keep you on track with your diet. Using a slow cooker and doubling or tripling the recipe allows you to make large batches . . . some to eat now, and some later, when you don't have time to cook.

Slow cookers also bring a depth of flavor to foods as the slow cooking process helps flavors slowly unfold, and supports the rich caramelization of meats and vegetables. Stirring in fresh ingredients at the very end adds complexity to the dish, and the moist cooking environment keeps meats rich and succulent.

If you haven't incorporated slow cooking into your Paleo routine, this is your invitation to start. The flavors of the food, and sheer convenience, will leave you wondering how you ever lived without this wonderful cooking technique.

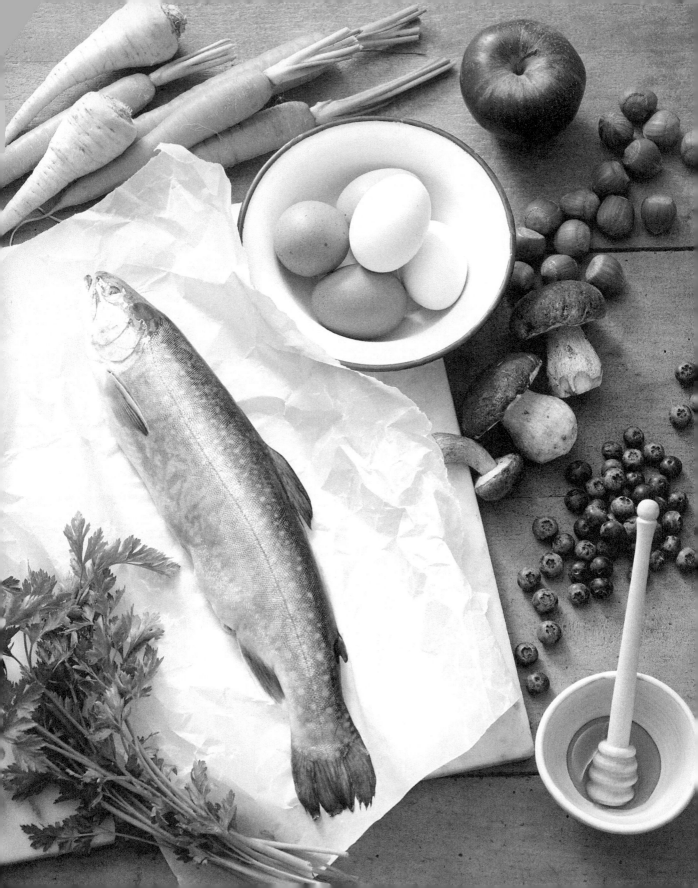

THE COMPLETE PALEO SLOW COOKER

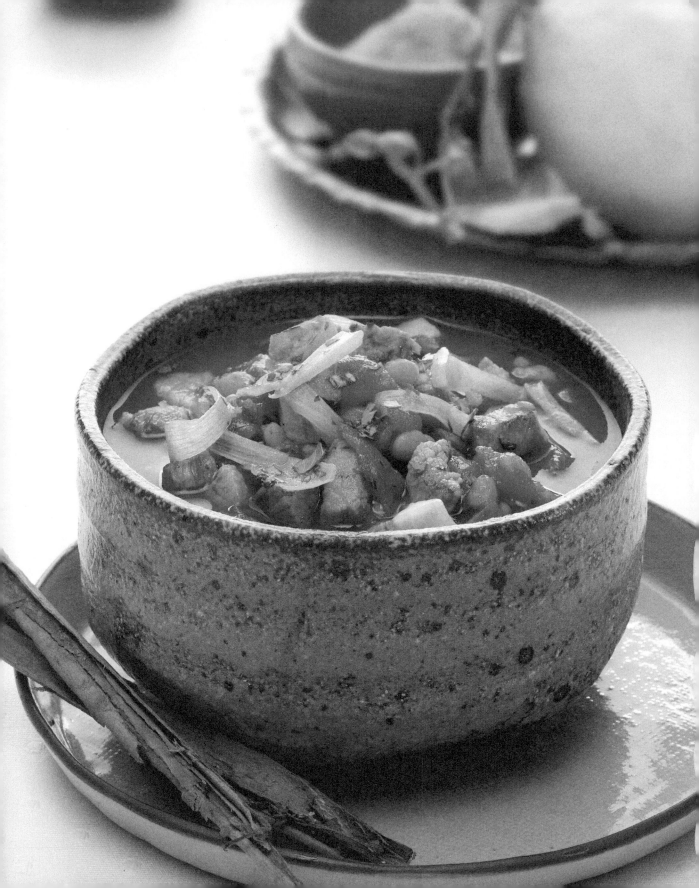

The Complete Paleo Slow Cooker

A Paleo Cookbook for Everyday
Meals That Prep Fast & Cook Slow

KAREN FRAZIER

**ROCKRIDGE
PRESS**

The Paleo Slow Cooker at a Glance

If you're looking for fast, easy, delicious and healthy meals that fit your Paleo lifestyle, this is the book for you. With more than 150 recipes that are fast and easy to prepare in your slow cooker, this cookbook makes the Paleo diet easier than ever.

The recipes in this book:

- Are full of Paleo-friendly, healthy ingredients
- Require fewer than 20 minutes of active prep time
- Contain easy-to-find ingredients
- Are "set and forget" recipes—you prepare them and they are ready eight to ten hours later; if the recipes do require you to add ingredients at the end, they are added within the last half-hour of cooking

Recipes may have one of two labels: Lower Sodium, meaning the recipe contains less than 300mg of sodium per serving, or Super Quick Prep, indicating that the recipe requires 10 minutes or less of active time.

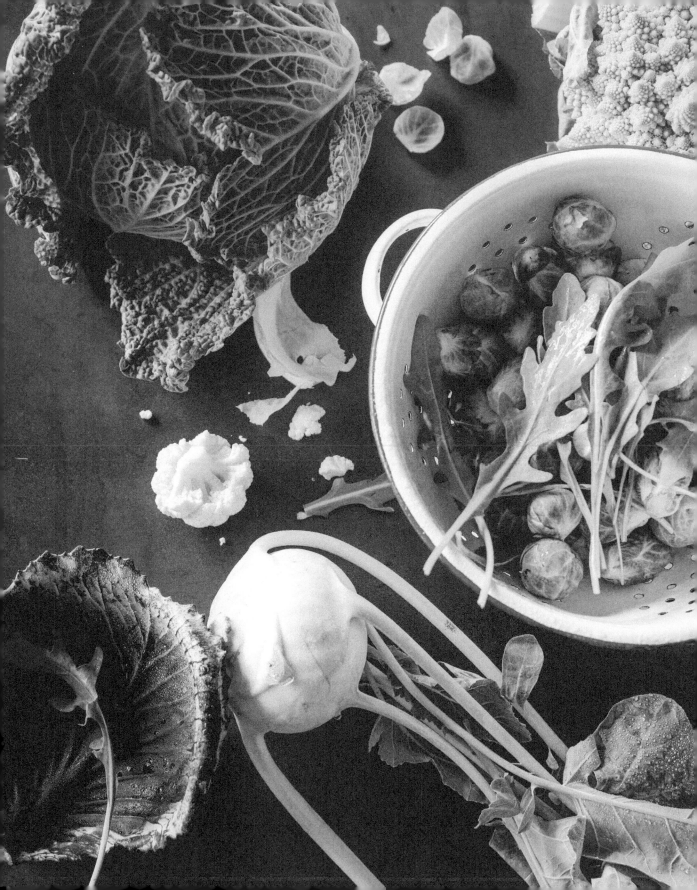

Contents

Introduction

SLOW COOKERS ARE FANTASTIC TIME-SAVING DEVICES, especially for people on eating plans like the Paleo diet who prepare mostly fresh foods for every meal. Using a slow cooker to prepare Paleo meals will save you time and provide you delicious, nutritious foods that fit your busy Paleo lifestyle.

For many people, one of the discouraging aspects of the Paleo diet is the amount of time spent preparing food. Since the majority of Paleo meals are made from scratch, many people prepare meals two or three times a day—which can take up a lot of prep and cooking time. Using a slow cooker strategically can help you minimize the time spent in your kitchen while still providing meals that taste great and meet your Paleo nutritional requirements.

Slow cookers are an excellent tool for preparing healthy Paleo meals because they require minimal prep time in the morning. You chop vegetables, add meat and some seasonings, put on the lid, and turn on the slow cooker. While you go about your busy day your slow cooker does the rest, magically blending and building flavors and providing you with hot, hearty, flavorful meals.

Some slow cooker recipes are less than convenient, though, because they have a lot of steps, require frequent supervision, and ask you to add ingredients at different intervals during the cooking process. This defeats the "set it and forget it" purpose of using a slow cooker. To create maximum convenience for people with busy lives, the recipes in this cookbook allow you to prepare and add your ingredients all at once and then walk away for several hours without doing anything else. If additional ingredients are required, you add them within the last 30 minutes of the cooking time. These late additions create additional flavor development, as you stir in fragrant herbs and incorporate ingredients to bring crispness or freshness to the dish. Still, even when recipes do call for these additions at the end of cooking, your total active time preparing each dish in this book is 20 minutes or less. You can save even more time by using precut vegetables.

Want to save even more kitchen time? Cook once, eat twice (or more). Cooking enough so you have leftovers for a second meal—to put in the freezer for meals on the go, or to reheat for breakfast or lunch the next day—saves you time and helps

CHAPTER ONE

The Many Health Benefits of a Slowly Cooked Paleo Diet

THE IDEA BEHIND THE PALEO DIET is to simplify the foods people eat, focusing on natural, whole ingredients that would have been available to our hunter-gatherer ancestors. This means the diet steers clear of many of the foods typically found in the traditional Western diet, such as processed foods with long lists of ingredients, highly processed industrial seed oils, grains, sugars, chemical additives, and factory-farmed animal products. Instead, the diet focuses on natural, whole foods, such as:

- Pastured (grass-fed) meats and poultry, including organ meats
- Organic fruits and vegetables
- Expeller-pressed virgin oils, such as olive oil, coconut oil, and avocado oil
- Eggs from pastured poultry
- Wild-caught seafood
- Natural sweeteners, like honey and maple syrup
- Organic nuts and seeds
- Herbs, spices, vinegars, and other natural flavoring agents, such as citrus zest and sea salt

Some recipes in this book have very low levels of salt or are especially quick to prepare. You'll see them labeled this way.

LS Lower Sodium: Contains less than 300mg of sodium per serving

QP Super Quick Prep: Takes 10 minutes or less of active time

SIX BENEFITS OF EATING PALEO

Eating a Paleo-style diet has a number of health benefits, many of which documented:

Promotes Weight Loss

Many people report losing weight on the Paleo diet, and science agrees. A study published in the March 2014 issue of *European Journal of Clinical Nutrition* looked at obese post-menopausal women. The two-year trial put women into two groups: one following a Paleo-style diet and the other following the Nordic Nutrition Recommendations. The women on the Paleo-style diet had greater fat and weight loss than those in the other group.

Improves Cardiac Risk Factors

Many factors correlate with an increased risk of developing cardiovascular and coronary artery disease, including high cholesterol, high triglycerides, and poor glycemic control. A randomized controlled study published in the July 2009 issue of *Cardiovascular Diabetology* compared patients on a Paleo-style diet with those on a standard diabetes diet. Another study reported in the August 2009 *European Journal of Clinical Nutrition* compared two groups without diabetes. In both studies, the people on the Paleo diet experienced lowered cardiac risk factors, including blood pressure, triglycerides, and blood cholesterol levels, and they exhibited better glycemic control.

Improves Metabolic Markers

People with metabolic syndrome, a cluster of symptoms that increases the risk of heart disease, stroke, and diabetes, experience improvement on a Paleo-style diet. Along with other symptoms, they have a specific pattern of fat distribution that seems to affect metabolic syndrome. A study published in the July 2013 issue of the *Journal of Internal Medicine* showed that following a Paleo diet affected how this fat was distributed, which improved insulin sensitivity, decreased liver fat, and led to overall fat loss. This change in fat distribution also decreased the risks associated with metabolic syndrome.

Decreases Inflammation

Inflammation plays a key role in numerous health issues, such as heart disease, chronic pain, and autoimmune diseases. According to Harvard Health Publications, a website run by the Harvard Medical School, the key to fighting inflammation lies in the foods you eat. Inflammatory foods (those that contribute to chronic inflammation) include refined carbohydrates (such as sugar, bread, and pasta), soda, and margarine. The Paleo diet eliminates these.

Likewise, foods rich in Omega-6 fatty acids tend to be inflammatory, while those rich in omega-3 fatty acids tend to be anti-inflammatory. The standard Western diet has a ratio of omega-6 to omega-3 fatty acids of about 15 to 1, while the actual ratio should be closer to 2 to 1, or even 1 to 1, according to an article in the October 2002 issue of *Biomedicine & Pharmacotherapy*. Balancing these ratios is critical to improving health, and the Paleo diet tends to have this ratio naturally under control.

Is Nutrient-Dense

The standard Western diet contains many foods that are high in calories but low in vitamins and minerals. The whole, natural foods on a Paleo diet, however, pack high levels of nutrients into every calorie. Therefore, this diet is a rich source of the micro- and macro-nutrients the body needs to perform daily functions.

Curbs Cravings

One of the best ways to improve your health through diet is to cut out junk foods, like fast food, sugars, sodas, baked goods, candy, and artificial ingredients. Sugar (and foods that break down quickly into simple sugars, such as refined carbohydrates) is a highly addictive substance that can cause significant cravings, according to MIT News, the website of the Massachusetts Institute of Technology. Because the Paleo diet cuts out refined carbs and sugar, you may experience less craving for sugary foods.

PALEO CAN BE VERSATILE

The list of foods that you can eat on a Paleo diet varies depending on who you talk to. The core diet consists of the foods on the very first page of this chapter, but there is room to add foods that may not be traditionally considered Paleo by strict adherents. Fortunately, there is some wiggle room, depending on how these foods affect your body. Such optional choices include:

- Dairy products from grass-fed animals (including grass-fed butter)
- Ghee
- White potatoes
- Alcohol

While the name "Paleo" seems to indicate you must only eat foods that were available to cave dwellers, what really matters is whether the foods are healthy for *you*. Therefore, it is possible to sometimes add certain ingredients that, while not strictly Paleo, aren't going to be harmful. For example, vinegar isn't strictly Paleo (it wasn't around at the time), but it is a naturally fermented product. Use your best judgment here; if you are sensitive to dairy products, for instance, chances are it's best to exclude grass-fed organic dairy, butter, or ghee from your diet. However, you may be able to have a little and be okay. In general, many people on a Paleo diet adhere to a 90/10 principle: If you eat strictly Paleo 90 percent of the time, you have 10 percent wiggle room.

Only a couple of the recipes in this book contain dairy, alcohol, or similar non-Paleo ingredients, and you can easily leave out and replace those with an ingredient that works for you. Likewise, some of the recipe notes offer a suggestion for adding a less Paleo ingredient (like grass-fed dairy) which you can add if your body tolerates it.

COOKING PALEO

While the Paleo diet is often thought of as the caveman diet, this doesn't mean you need to cook everything over an open flame or on a heated rock, as your ancestors would have. Although cooking over an open flame (or in a smoker or on a grill or barbecue for modern cave dwellers) can yield some superbly delicious results, and is wholeheartedly encouraged, it's not always practical. Most days probably you just don't have the time, energy, attention, or patience to carefully tend meat and vegetables over a flame—not even a stovetop. That's why the modern cave dweller needs more cooking tools at his disposal.

Fortunately, in modern times there are plenty of other ways to quickly prepare a delicious Paleo meal. And at the top of the heap for the busy modern cave dweller is the slow cooker. It is the perfect cooking method when your life is just a little crazy and you're constantly rushing to meet the demands of your family, work, hobbies, exercise routine, community involvement, and all the other pressures of modern day life that keep you on the move.

In fact, if you're living a Paleo lifestyle and have other things going on in your life as well (and who doesn't?), then a slow cooker is a must. You'll be glad to know you've got a hot meal on the way when you're in the midst of your crazy day, and preparing the food will only require a minimal time commitment. A slow cooker is also an excellent way to keep you on plan. You can prepare extra meals in the slow cooker to freeze, so that when you don't have the time or energy to cook, you can pop a premade meal out of the freezer and heat it up—instead of heading for your nearest fast food joint.

For the recipes in this book, a six-quart slow cooker is a good choice, as it fits large cuts of meat and also allows you to double recipes or cook a little extra, giving you a few more meals you won't need to worry about.

SLOW COOKING DONE PALEO

Commercial slow cookers have been around since the 1970s, and they have always proved popular. Sales slowed down a little when microwave ovens became fashionable, but the microwave can never cook like a slow cooker. Slow cooking can benefit your food in many ways:

It Keeps Foods Moist

The closed environment of your slow cooker will keep meats moist and tender, particularly if they are high in fat or if you add a little broth. The lid and the low heat prevent moisture from evaporating into the air, keeping it in your food.

It Keeps Meat Very Tender

According to Science of Cooking, when you cook meat in a slow cooker at a low temperature, it breaks down the collagen in the meat, making it very tender as it cooks over a long period.

SLOW COOKER HEALTH HAZARDS

In general, slow cookers allow you to make healthy foods safely, but there are a few risks to be aware of:

DRIED BEAN TOXINS While this isn't an issue if you are Paleo (because you don't eat beans), it's important to note that cooking dried beans in a slow cooker can release toxins called "phytohemagglutinin." To prevent this, boil the beans over high heat for 10 minutes on the stovetop before transferring them to a slow cooker.

LEAD According to Paleo Leap, the crock of some slow cookers may contain lead and cadmium in the glazing, which has the potential to leach into food. As long as the glaze isn't scratched or cracked, this is not likely to be an issue. However, if there are scratches or chips, replace the crock. You can also buy slow cookers without lead in the glaze.

FOOD SAFETY When you don't keep foods hot enough, they can grow bacteria rapidly. WebMD suggests not using any frozen foods in your slow cooker (which can cause the foods to heat too slowly), cutting meat into smaller chunks, and starting the first hour on high before turning it to low if ingredients are very cold, to bring everything to a simmer more quickly.

NUTRIENT LOSS? While some people are concerned that cooking low and slow destroys vitamins and minerals, nutrition and natural health expert Dr. Andrew Weil suggests slow cooking does not destroy nutrients but rather preserves them to create healthy, vitamin- and mineral-rich meals.

It Can Save You Money

Pastured animal products tend to be costlier than their factory-farmed counterparts. However, because of the way slow cooking affects collagen in meat, it provides an excellent method for cooking less expensive cuts of meat, which lend themselves well to stewing. While the slow cooker isn't ideal for an expensive cut, such as a prime rib roast or beef tenderloin, it can work wonders on tenderizing a tough, cheap cut of chuck.

You Can Take Food with You

If you've ever gone to a potluck as a Paleo dieter, you've probably discovered that there aren't a whole lot of people who bring Paleo-friendly dishes to share. Enter the slow cooker, which allows you to make a Paleo-friendly meal and then transport it in the same convenient container. It's great for bringing food to share anywhere you know there won't be any Paleo-friendly foods. It can keep you on track, even when you're faced with tempting treats.

KNOW YOUR SLOW COOKER

If you're new to slow cooking, you may be a bit nervous about doing it right. Fortunately, slow cooking is relatively foolproof, as long as you keep a few tips in mind:

Cooking Temperatures

Slow cookers come in a few different varieties. The basic slow cooker has a simple temperature dial with three settings: low, high, and keep warm. Fancier slow cookers may have programmable settings, which you can set to cook on high for a certain period, cook on low for a certain period, and then keep warm until you are ready to eat. While either type is effective, the programmable ones may be best for you if you truly want to set it and forget it, because you can program exactly the amount of time you want at each stage, and ensure a perfectly cooked meal when you get home. However, if you plan to cook your food for eight to ten hours, then a basic slow cooker set on low will be just fine.

Cooking Time

A slow cooker's low and high settings are very different from your stovetop. High on your stovetop will cook food in a matter of minutes. In a slow cooker, it will take several hours. Slow cooking is named that way for a reason: you're not going to have a meal cooked and on the table in 30 minutes using this appliance. The process is slow. Standard cooking times are typically about three to five hours on high, or eight to ten hours on low.

Shape and Size

Slow cookers come in a range of shapes and sizes. The recipes in this cookbook are designed for a six-quart slow cooker. You can choose a smaller slow cooker, but you may need to halve the recipes. Oblong slow cookers are best for fitting roasts and whole chickens, so this is probably your best choice.

Adjusting to Your Slow Cooker Size

If you have a smaller or larger slow cooker, this book is still right for you. You don't need to go out and buy a six-quart oblong one—unless you've been looking for an excuse to buy a new toy. Slow cooking is an inexact science, and it works beautifully even if you dump and eyeball ingredient amounts. If your slow cooker is a different size:

- Halve recipes or double them.
- Trim whole cuts of meat to fit your slow cooker, or cut into bite-size pieces.
- Add fewer or more veggies.

- Add less or more liquid.
- Don't fill your slow cooker more than three-quarters full, or leave it less than half full.

SLOW COOKER TRICKS AND TIPS

To maximize success with your slow cooker, consider the following:

- DO put vegetables on the bottom and meat on the top. Then, pour liquid and seasonings over the top of the meat.
- DON'T preheat your slow cooker. Put the foods in the slow cooker, and then bring it up to temperature.
- DO add fresh herbs, citrus juice, or vinegars at the end of cooking, because they impart a bright, fresh flavor that's a nice contrast to the deep flavors developed during slow cooking.
- DON'T be afraid to use dried herbs and ingredients like garlic powder and onion powder. Fresh garlic is nice, but in a slow cooker it loses that fresh garlic flavor anyway. Garlic powder releases the same flavors after hours

of cooking, and it's a lot quicker to use than chopping fresh garlic. Choose organic herbs and spices, and make sure you read ingredients to make sure they don't contain any additives.

- DON'T leave out the salt. Sea salt and Himalayan pink salt are great choices for Paleo cooking. Salt is essential for flavor development. The recipes in this book call for sea salt, which has minerals in it that make it slightly more nutritious than table salt.

- DON'T add hot vegetables to cold meats, which can encourage bacteria growth. If you precook veggies to add to the slow cooker, you also need to prebrown the meat.

- DO add extra liquid if the meat you're using looks relatively low in fat. Grass-fed meats are often lower in fat and may require a bit of extra liquid. A cup of stock or a few tablespoons of animal fat, such as duck fat or lard, are good choices.

- DON'T lift the lid and keep checking on your food. This lets steam and heat escape, which can dry out food and encourage bacteria growth. Instead, put the lid on, turn it on, and just walk away.

- DO cut vegetable chunks to about the same size so they cook evenly. If you're cutting your meat, cut it into similar size chunks, as well.

- DON'T reheat in your slow cooker, as it won't get hot enough for leftovers and could allow foodborne bacteria to grow. Reheat on the stovetop or in the microwave.

- DON'T store leftover food in the slow cooker insert, as this may damage the crock. Transfer it to appropriate airtight containers and refrigerate right away.

- DON'T stir the dish unless instructed to in the recipe. This can dry out food and encourage bacteria growth.

- DON'T wash your slow cooker insert with an abrasive sponge, which can scratch the crock.

- DON'T fill it all the way to the top, particularly with liquid. While a roast may touch the top of the slow cooker, it will shrink as it cooks. If you're cooking a soup, however, you don't want the slow cooker to be more than three-quarters full (or less than half full).

- DON'T add frozen foods to the slow cooker. This can prevent the temperature from rising quickly enough, which can encourage bacteria growth.

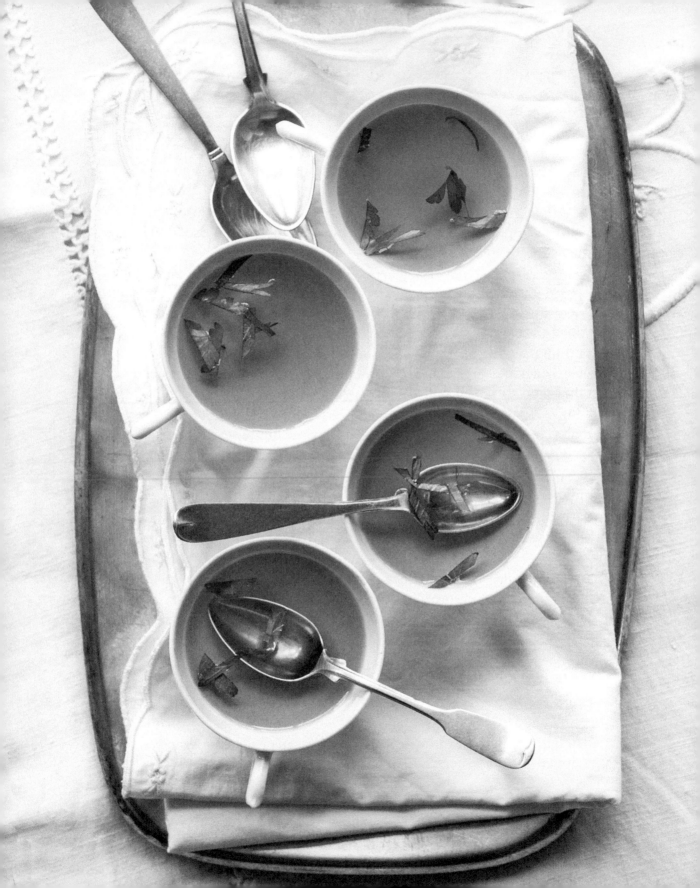

Stocks, Broths, and Sauces

Vegetable Stock

PREP TIME: 5 MINUTES / COOK TIME: 8 TO 12 HOURS

QP

MAKES ABOUT 10 CUPS With your slow cooker, making homemade stocks and broths has never been easier, or more hands-off. You can flavor this tasty stock with any veggies and herbs you like, so feel free to branch out the recipe. Stock is also a great way to use veggie trimmings. When you use vegetables in other dishes, fill a zip-top bag with trimmings and peels from onions, celery, carrots, fennel, mushrooms, garlic, and fresh herbs (avoid super-strong veggies like cruciferous vegetables or peppers). Keep the trimmings in your freezer, and when you're ready to make stock, just dump a gallon-size bag of trimmings into the slow cooker and cover it with water.

2 celery stalks (leaves included), quartered

4 ounces mushrooms (stems included)

2 carrots (unpeeled), quartered

1 onion (unpeeled), quartered pole to pole

1 garlic head (unpeeled), halved across the middle

2 fresh thyme sprigs

10 peppercorns

½ teaspoon sea salt

Water to fill the slow cooker three-quarters full

1. In the slow cooker, combine the celery, mushrooms, carrots, onion, garlic, thyme, peppercorns, salt, and water.

2. Cover and simmer on low for 8 to 12 hours.

3. Strain the stock through a fine-mesh sieve, and discard the solids.

4. Store the stock in a tightly sealed container in the refrigerator for up to 5 days, or in the freezer for up to a year.

PRECOOKING: If you want to get more flavor from your veggies in the stock, roast them in a 450°F oven for about 30 minutes before adding them to the slow cooker.

PER SERVING (1 CUP) CALORIES: 38; PROTEIN: 5G; CARBOHYDRATES: 1G; FAT: 0G; FIBER: 0G; SUGAR: 1G; SODIUM: 350MG

Mushroom Stock

PREP TIME: 5 MINUTES / COOK TIME: 8 TO 12 HOURS

(QP)

MAKES ABOUT 10 CUPS If you enjoy the earthy flavor of mushrooms, this broth is for you. It's wonderful for sipping by itself, or it makes a great base for stews. For a quick meal, you can sauté some veggies and meat in a small pot and add the stock for a hearty soup. The dried mushrooms really pump up the flavor, and they're easy to find in the bulk foods or produce section of your local grocery store. If you can't find dried porcini mushrooms, feel free to substitute with any type of dry mushrooms you can find.

1 onion (unpeeled), quartered pole to pole

2 carrots (unpeeled), quartered

2 celery stalks, quartered

1 garlic head (unpeeled), halved across the middle

8 ounces fresh cremini mushrooms

2 ounces dried porcini mushrooms

1 teaspoon dried thyme or 2 fresh thyme sprigs

10 peppercorns

½ teaspoon sea salt

Water to fill the slow cooker three-quarters full

1. In the slow cooker, combine the onion, carrots, celery, garlic, mushrooms, thyme, peppercorns, salt, and water

2. Cover and simmer on low for 8 to 12 hours.

3. Strain the stock through a fine-mesh sieve, and discard the solids.

4. Store the stock in a tightly sealed container in the refrigerator for up to 5 days, or in the freezer for up to a year.

PRECOOKING: Try roasting the garlic before adding it to the stock. Wrap the garlic in foil and put it in a 350°F oven for 90 minutes, or follow the Roasted Garlic recipe (page 33). Roasting the garlic adds deep caramel notes to the earthy mushroom broth.

PER SERVING (1 CUP) CALORIES: 38; PROTEIN: 5G; CARBOHYDRATES: 1G; FAT: 0G; FIBER: 0G; SUGAR: 1G; SODIUM: 350MG

Fish Stock

PREP TIME: 5 MINUTES / COOK TIME: 8 TO 12 HOURS

QP

MAKES ABOUT 10 CUPS Fish stock has a delicate flavor that's perfect for chowders and seafood stews. You can use fish bones from halibut, haddock, flounder, bass, or sole, or shells from shrimp, crab, or lobster. For stronger flavor, add one or two fish heads from cod or haddock. Before adding the bones, rinse them clean of blood. Trim any gills from the heads before adding. To avoid having to buy fish bones, whenever you cook fish or peel crustaceans, save the bones and shells in a zip-top bag in your freezer for the next time you make stock.

2 to 3 pounds bones from white fish and/or crustacean shells

1 to 2 fish heads from white fish (optional)

1 carrot, roughly chopped

1 celery stalk (leaves included), roughly chopped

1 onion, roughly chopped

2 dried bay leaves

2 fresh thyme sprigs or 1 teaspoon dried thyme

8 peppercorns

½ teaspoon sea salt

Water to fill the slow cooker three-quarters full

1. In the slow cooker, combine the fish bones, fish heads (if using), carrot, celery, onion, bay leaves, thyme, peppercorns, salt, and water.

2. Cover and simmer on low for 8 to 12 hours.

3. Strain the stock through a fine-mesh sieve, and discard the solids.

4. Cover the broth, and refrigerate for 2 to 3 hours.

5. Using a spoon, remove the fat that has solidified on the stock's surface. Discard the fat.

6. Store the stock in a tightly sealed container in the refrigerator for up to 5 days, or in the freezer for up to a year.

A LITTLE LESS PALEO: Add a delicate wine flavor to the broth by stirring in a half cup of dry white wine, such as Chardonnay or Chenin Blanc, 30 minutes before you are done cooking. Leave the lid off for the remaining 30 minutes.

PER SERVING (1 CUP) CALORIES: 38; PROTEIN: 5G; CARBOHYDRATES: 1G; FAT: 0G; FIBER: 0G; SUGAR: 1G; SODIUM: 350MG

Ginger-Poultry Broth

PREP TIME: 5 MINUTES / COOK TIME: 12 TO 24 HOURS

QP

MAKES ABOUT 10 CUPS This Asia-inspired broth has the bright bite of ginger over the deeper flavors of chicken or turkey. Extra garlic also ups the flavor, making this an excellent base for all sorts of Asian soups and stews. The warming broth is also great for sipping when you have a cold or the flu, as the heat of the ginger and garlic can help clear out your sinuses.

2 pounds chicken wings, backs, or feet

2 garlic heads (unpeeled), halved across the middle

1 (2-inch) ginger knob (unpeeled), cut into ¼-inch-thick slices

1 carrot (unpeeled), halved

1 celery stalk (unpeeled), halved

12 peppercorns

½ teaspoon sea salt

Water to cover all the ingredients

1. In the slow cooker, combine the chicken wings, garlic, ginger, carrot, celery, peppercorns, salt, and water.

2. Cover and simmer on low for 12 to 24 hours. Don't go past 24 hours, or the broth may become bitter.

3. Strain the broth through a fine-mesh sieve, and discard the solids.

4. Refrigerate the broth, covered, for 2 hours.

5. Using a spoon, remove the fat that has solidified on the stock's surface. Discard the fat or save it for cooking later.

6. Store the broth in a tightly sealed container in the refrigerator for up to 5 days, or in the freezer for up to a year.

> **NUTRITION HIGHLIGHT:** Ginger is well-known for it's healing power. It's commonly used to ease gastro-intestinal distress, and it is also anti-inflammatory, according to the World's Healthiest Foods website.

PER SERVING (1 CUP) CALORIES: 38; PROTEIN: 5G; CARBOHYDRATES: 1G; FAT: 0G; FIBER: 0G; SUGAR: 1G; SODIUM: 350MG

Bone Broth
(Poultry, Pork, Lamb, or Beef)

PREP TIME: 5 MINUTES / COOK TIME: 12 TO 24 HOURS

QP

MAKES ABOUT 6 CUPS Richly flavored, bone broth adds a deep savoriness to your soups and stews. It is miles ahead of the canned broth you find at the grocery store, and you have complete control over the ingredients. Best of all, you can use poultry, pork, lamb, or beef bones in the broth, and they can be reused once or twice to make more broth, so it's economical too. You control the salt level, and you can change the flavor profile by using different herbs, adding mushrooms, or changing the vegetables you use.

2 to 3 pounds poultry, pork, lamb, or beef bones

1 garlic head (unpeeled), halved across the middle

1 onion (unpeeled), quartered pole to pole

2 carrots (unpeeled), halved

2 celery stalks (unpeeled), halved

1 tablespoon apple cider vinegar

2 dried bay leaves

2 fresh rosemary sprigs or 1 teaspoon dried rosemary

2 fresh thyme sprigs or 1 teaspoon dried thyme

10 peppercorns

½ teaspoon sea salt

Water to cover all the ingredients

1. In the slow cooker, combine the bones, garlic, onion, carrots, celery, vinegar, bay leaves, rosemary, thyme, peppercorns, salt, and water.

2. Cover and simmer on low for 12 to 24 hours. For beef, lamb, and pork bones, you can cook as long as 48 hours. For poultry bones, keep the cooking time to 24 hours or less.

3. Strain the broth through a fine-mesh sieve, reserving the bones for another use (if you like) and discarding the vegetable and herb solids.

4. Cover the broth and refrigerate for 2 hours.

5. Using a spoon, remove the fat that has solidified on the stock's surface. Discard the fat or save it for cooking later.

6. Store the stock in a tightly sealed container in the refrigerator for up to 5 days, or in the freezer for up to a year.

NUTRITION HIGHLIGHT: Bone broth is a highly nourishing food. The long hours of cooking pull minerals from the bones, which can support your health. Cartilage in the bones also creates gelatin, which gives the broth body, and is beneficial to your joints and gut healing, according to Paleo Leap.

PER SERVING (1 CUP) CALORIES: 38; PROTEIN: 5G; CARBOHYDRATES: 1G; FAT: 0G; FIBER: 0G; SUGAR: 1G; SODIUM: 350MG

Orange-Chili-Garlic Sauce

PREP TIME: 15 MINUTES / COOK TIME: 8 HOURS

MAKES ABOUT 5 CUPS Sriracha is a spicy, garlicky sauce that adds a punch of heat and lots of flavor to your foods. Unfortunately, traditional store-bought sriracha isn't quite Paleo—it has sugar in it, which is something you definitely want to avoid. This Paleo slow cooker version of sriracha will fill your house with the spicy fragrance of citrus and chiles as it cooks, and it makes a delicious addition to any food to which you'd like to add some heat. It's spicy, slightly sweet, and has a nice bit of acid, as well. For safety, wear gloves when you chop the peppers, and keep your fingers away from your eyes!

½ cup apple cider vinegar

4 pounds red jalapeño peppers, stems, seeds, and ribs removed, chopped

10 garlic cloves, chopped

½ cup tomato paste

Juice and zest of 1 orange

½ cup honey

2 tablespoons Asian fish sauce (try a Paleo-friendly blend, such as Red Boat) or coconut aminos

2 teaspoons sea salt

1. In the slow cooker, combine the vinegar, peppers, garlic, tomato paste, orange juice and zest, honey, fish sauce, and salt.

2. Cover and simmer on low for 8 hours.

3. Store the sauce in a tightly sealed container in the refrigerator for up to 1 month, or in the freezer for up to a year.

PORTION ADJUSTMENT: If you like your food hot and go through a lot of spicy sauces like sriracha, you can make a larger batch by doubling or tripling the recipe, because this sauce freezes well. You can also halve the batch if you have a smaller slow cooker.

PER SERVING (2 TABLESPOONS) CALORIES: 33; PROTEIN: 1G; CARBOHYDRATES: 8G; SUGAR: 6G; FAT: <1G; FIBER: 2G; SODIUM: 167MG

Cooked Salsa

PREP TIME: 20 MINUTES / COOK TIME: 8 HOURS

(LS)

MAKES ABOUT 5 CUPS Homemade salsa with onions, garlic, chiles, and spices adds flavor to foods, and it's a perfect topper for meat in tacos and tasty with eggs. This cooked version freezes well, so you can make a big batch and keep it in your freezer, tightly sealed, for up to one year. Feel free to adjust the seasonings to your taste.

3 onions, chopped

8 jalapeño peppers, seeds, stems, and ribs removed, chopped

2 pounds roma tomatoes (whole)

2 (28-ounce) cans stewed tomatoes, drained

8 garlic cloves, minced

Juice of 2 limes

½ cup chopped fresh cilantro

1 teaspoon sea salt

1. In the slow cooker, combine the onions and jalapeños with the fresh and canned tomatoes.

2. Cover and cook on low for 8 hours.

3. Stir in the garlic, lime juice, cilantro, and salt.

4. Using a potato masher, mash the salsa, or purée in a blender or food processor.

5. Store the salsa in a tightly sealed container in the refrigerator for up to 1 week, or in the freezer for up to a year.

A LITTLE LESS PALEO: Add a boozy hit to your salsa by adding ¼ cup to ½ cup of tequila to the slow cooker at the start of cooking.

PER SERVING (2 TABLESPOONS) CALORIES: 23; PROTEIN: 1G; CARBOHYDRATES: 5G; SUGAR: 3G; FAT: <1G; FIBER: 2G; SODIUM: 45MG

Gravy

PREP TIME: 10 MINUTES / COOK TIME: 8 HOURS

MAKES ABOUT 6 CUPS Looking for a thick, rich gravy to serve with meats? This version adds the fresh flavor of herbs, and it's really easy to make. Traditional gravy relies on wheat flour (or other grain-based starches) to thicken it. This one uses the starch from carrots, which adds a sweetness and flavor you can't find in other gravies.

4 cups Bone Broth, plus more if
    needed (page 26)

1 onion, chopped

1 pound carrots, peeled and chopped

8 ounces whole mushrooms

1 teaspoon garlic powder

1 teaspoon dried thyme

1 teaspoon dried rosemary

1 teaspoon dried mustard powder or
    1 tablespoon Dijon mustard

1 teaspoon sea salt

¼ teaspoon freshly ground black pepper

1. In the slow cooker, combine the Bone Broth, onion, carrots, mushrooms, garlic powder, thyme, rosemary, mustard powder, salt, and pepper.

2. Cover and cook on low for 8 hours.

3. Using a slotted spoon, transfer all the vegetables to a blender or food processor, or put them in a bowl and use a potato masher or immersion blender. Purée the vegetables until smooth.

4. Return the vegetables to the liquid, and stir to combine, adding more Bone Broth if needed to adjust the thickness of the gravy.

5. Store the gravy in a tightly sealed container in the refrigerator for up to 5 days, or in the freezer for up to a year.

> **A LITTLE LESS PALEO:** Replace 2 cups of the Bone Broth with 2 cups of a dry red wine, such as Syrah or Cabernet Sauvignon, for a richer flavor.

PER SERVING (¼ CUP) CALORIES: 19; PROTEIN: 1G; CARBOHYDRATES: 3G; SUGAR: 1G; FAT: <1G; FIBER: 1G; SODIUM: 219MG

Marinara Sauce

PREP TIME: 10 MINUTES / COOK TIME: 8 HOURS

MAKES ABOUT 6 CUPS Marinara is a classic Italian red sauce that has lots of rich tomato, garlic, and herb flavors. This version doubles up on the flavor, with dried herbs at the start of cooking and fresh basil stirred in at the end. This freezes well, so you can make a big batch and use it as a topping for meats, veggie noodles, or eggs.

2 pounds roma tomatoes (leave them whole)

1 (28-ounce) can stewed tomatoes, drained

1 (6-ounce) can tomato paste

2 teaspoons garlic powder

2 tablespoons Italian seasoning

2 dried bay leaves

2 tablespoons honey

2 tablespoons balsamic vinegar

¼ teaspoon crushed red pepper flakes

1 teaspoon sea salt

½ teaspoon freshly ground black pepper

½ cup chopped fresh basil

1. In the slow cooker, combine the fresh and canned tomatoes, tomato paste, garlic powder, Italian seasoning, bay leaves, honey, balsamic vinegar, red pepper flakes, salt, and pepper.

2. Cover and cook on low for 8 hours.

3. Remove the bay leaves. Stir in the basil, using the spoon to lightly mash the tomatoes.

4. Store the marinara sauce in a tightly sealed container in the refrigerator for up to 5 days or in the freezer for up to 1 year.

NUTRITION HIGHLIGHT: Tomatoes are rich in lycopene, an antioxidant that has been shown to aid in preventing certain cancers, according to the Mayo Clinic.

PER SERVING (½ CUP) CALORIES: 58; PROTEIN: 2G; CARBOHYDRATES: 12G; SUGAR: 9G; FAT: 1G; FIBER: 2G; SODIUM: 178MG

Meat Sauce (Bolognese)

PREP TIME: 15 MINUTES / COOK TIME: 8 HOURS

MAKES ABOUT 5 CUPS Bolognese sauce is rich, meaty, and fragrant with herbs. It's a perfect topper for spaghetti squash, sweet potatoes, or homemade cauliflower rice (simply pulse cauliflower in a food processor, or grate it and sauté in a little olive oil for about 5 minutes). This version cooks all day in a slow cooker, giving the flavors time to blend and develop into a rich, tasty meat sauce. This freezes well for up to one year in a tightly sealed container.

3 onions, finely chopped

1 pound ground grass-fed beef, crumbled

1 pound ground pastured pork, crumbled

¼ cup tomato paste

1 cup unsweetened almond milk

2 teaspoons dried oregano

2 teaspoons dried basil

2 teaspoons garlic powder

1 teaspoon sea salt

¼ teaspoon crushed red pepper flakes

¼ teaspoon freshly ground black pepper

1. In the slow cooker, combine the onions, beef, pork, tomato paste, almond milk, oregano, basil, garlic, salt, red pepper flakes, and pepper.

2. Cover and cook on low for 8 hours.

3. Store the sauce in a tightly sealed container in the refrigerator for up to 5 days, or in the freezer for up to a year.

> **A LITTLE LESS PALEO:** Add ½ cup of red wine at the start of cooking to deepen the flavors. Just reduce the almond milk by ½ cup.

PER SERVING (½ CUP) CALORIES: 196; PROTEIN: 18G; CARBOHYDRATES: 4G; SUGAR: 2G; FAT: 12G; FIBER: 1G; SODIUM: 236MG

Roasted Garlic

PREP TIME: 10 MINUTES / COOK TIME: 4 TO 6 HOURS

(LS) (QP)

MAKES 8 TO 12 GARLIC BULBS Roasted garlic has a caramelized, mellow flavor that adds richness to many foods, including stocks and sauces. You can also mash roasted garlic cloves and spread them on meats, mix them with veggies, and use them to add flavor to just about any Paleo meal. This recipe makes several bulbs at once, so you can freeze the individual bulbs or cloves in zip-top bags for up to one year, or store them in the refrigerator for up to one week.

8 to 12 garlic bulbs (or however many fit to line the bottom of the slow cooker), tops chopped off so the cloves are exposed

½ cup extra-virgin olive oil, melted duck fat, or your favorite Paleo-friendly oil or fat

1 teaspoon sea salt

1. Place the garlic bulbs, cut-side up, so they line the bottom of the slow cooker.

1. Drizzle the bulbs with the oil, and sprinkle with the sea salt.

3. Cover and cook on low for 4 to 6 hours, or until the garlic cloves are browned and soft.

4. Store the roasted garlic in a tightly sealed container in the refrigerator for up to a week or in the freezer for up to a year. Reserve the garlic-flavored oil or fat for another cooking use, if you like.

> **NUTRITION HIGHLIGHT:** Garlic has many healthy properties, due largely to a compound it contains called "allicin." According to the Linus Pauling Institute, allicin may be beneficial in fighting a number of diseases.

PER SERVING (¼ CUP) CALORIES: 19; PROTEIN: 1G; CARBOHYDRATES: 3G; SUGAR: 1G; FAT: <1G; FIBER: 1G; SODIUM: 219MG

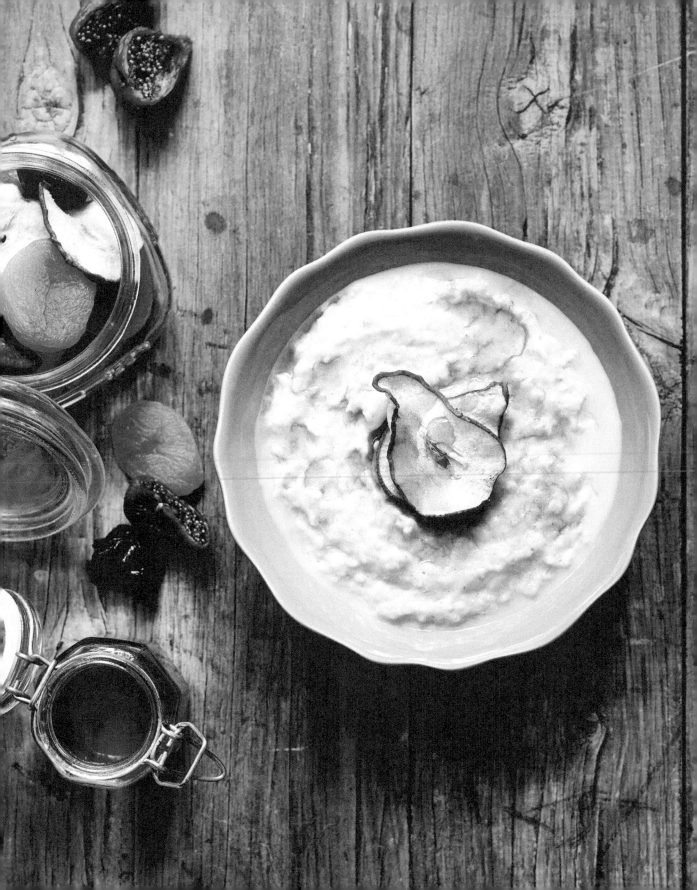

Breakfast and Brunch

Honey-Coconut Porridge

PREP TIME: 5 MINUTES / COOK TIME: 8 HOURS

SERVES 6 Porridge makes a hearty, nutritious breakfast. This sweet, hot breakfast has a light coconut flavor with a hint of honey. You can stir in your favorite chopped nuts or seeds for texture, or your favorite dried or fresh fruits; add them at the start or sprinkle them right into your bowl. Set this up to cook before you go to bed, and it will be ready first thing in the morning. It's a wonderfully tasty way to start your day.

4 cups light coconut milk

3 cups apple juice

2¼ cups coconut flour

1 teaspoon ground cinnamon

¼ cup honey

1. In the slow cooker, stir to combine the coconut milk, apple juice, coconut flour, cinnamon, and honey.

2. Cover and cook on low for 8 hours, and serve.

SEASONAL INGREDIENTS: Add in-season fresh fruits just before serving. For example, in June add a ¼ cup of sliced fresh strawberries, or add fresh blueberries in July and August. Plums or pluots are wonderful in late summer.

PER SERVING CALORIES: 372; PROTEIN: 8G; CARBOHYDRATES: 56G; SUGAR: 28G; FAT: 14G; FIBER: 15G; SODIUM: 134MG

Butternut Squash Porridge

PREP TIME: 10 MINUTES / COOK TIME: 8 HOURS

SERVES 6 Butternut squash has an earthy, sweet flavor that pairs beautifully with the spices and dried fruits in this tasty breakfast porridge. You can customize it by adding your own spice blends, or alternate between maple syrup and honey to add additional sweetness. It's a delicious, sweet, stick-to-your-ribs way to start your day.

2 butternut squash, skins and seeds removed, cut into 1-inch cubes

1 cup freshly squeezed orange juice

Zest of 1 orange

¼ cup pure maple syrup

1 teaspoon ground cinnamon

½ teaspoon ground ginger

½ teaspoon ground nutmeg

½ cup chopped pecans

1. In the slow cooker, combine the squash, orange juice, orange zest, maple syrup, cinnamon, ginger, and nutmeg.

2. Cover and cook on low for 8 hours.

3. Using a potato masher, mash the squash, or purée it in a blender or food processor.

4. Stir in the pecans, and serve.

> **NUTRITION HIGHLIGHT:** Butternut squash contains about 54 percent of your recommended daily intake of vitamin A. It's also rich in vitamins C and B6, and manganese.

PER SERVING CALORIES: 250; PROTEIN: 5G; CARBOHYDRATES: 24G; SUGAR: 15G; FAT: 14G; FIBER: 5G; SODIUM: 7MG

Sweet Potato Porridge WITH Vanilla, Cinnamon AND Cardamom

PREP TIME: 10 MINUTES / COOK TIME: 8 HOURS

SERVES 6 Sweet potatoes are earthy, sweet, and starchy, so they make a great breakfast mash. This version is fragrant with sweet spices, including cinnamon and cardamom, while vanilla adds a comforting, familiar flavor. You can adjust the flavors by replacing the coconut milk with fruit juice, such as orange or apple juice.

6 sweet potatoes, peeled and cut into 1-inch cubes

1½ cups light coconut milk

1 teaspoon ground cardamom

1 teaspoon ground cinnamon

1 teaspoon pure vanilla extract

1 cup raisins

Pinch sea salt

1. In the slow cooker, combine the sweet potatoes, coconut milk, cardamom, cinnamon, and vanilla.

2. Cover and cook on low for 8 hours.

3. Using a potato masher, mash the sweet potatoes and stir to combine with the liquid, or purée in a blender or food processor.

4. Stir in the raisins and salt, and serve.

NUTRITION HIGHLIGHT: Sweet potatoes are high in antioxidants, containing more than 100 percent of your recommended daily allowance of vitamin A. They are also an excellent source of vitamin C and manganese.

PER SERVING CALORIES: 317; PROTEIN: 4G; CARBOHYDRATES: 71G; SUGAR: 15G; FAT: 3G; FIBER: 8G; SODIUM: 73MG

Almond Meal WITH Dried Fruit Porridge

PREP TIME: 10 MINUTES / COOK TIME: 8 HOURS

SERVES 6 Dried fruits sweeten this delicious almond meal porridge. You can use any dried fruits you like—there's no need to stick to what's mentioned here. Honey sweetens the cereal, as does the apple cider. This is a hot breakfast that will carry you through your busy morning.

4 cups apple cider

3 cups almond meal

¼ cup honey

¼ cup dried apples

¼ cup dried apricots

¼ cup dried prunes

2 tablespoons coconut flour

1 teaspoon ground cinnamon

¼ teaspoon ground ginger

Pinch sea salt

1. In the slow cooker, combine the apple cider, almond meal, honey, dried fruits, coconut flour, cinnamon, ginger, and salt.

2. Cover and cook on low for 8 hours, and serve.

A LITTLE LESS PALEO: To make this cereal even richer, stir in ¼ cup of heavy cream just before serving. Sweeten it to taste with additional honey or maple syrup.

PER SERVING CALORIES: 430; PROTEIN: 1G; CARBOHYDRATES: 49G; SUGAR: 36G; FAT: 24G; FIBER: 8G; SODIUM: 39MG

Slow Cooker Breakfast Meatloaf

PREP TIME: 20 MINUTES / COOK TIME: 8 HOURS

SERVES 4 Try this tasty meatloaf for breakfast. Savory with the flavor of breakfast sausage and herbs, it's a protein-packed way to start your day. The best part is you don't need to buy premade breakfast sausage—you make it yourself by adding herbs and spices to ground pork. For an extra treat, try wrapping the meatloaf with thinly sliced bacon or pancetta before you cook it.

1 pound ground pork

1 cup almond meal

½ cup unsweetened almond milk

1 egg, beaten

1 onion, grated

1 carrot, grated

1 tablespoon coconut aminos

2 teaspoons dried sage

1 teaspoon garlic powder

1 teaspoon sea salt

¼ teaspoon freshly ground black pepper

Paleo-friendly fat or oil, for greasing

1. In a large bowl, mix together the pork, almond meal, almond milk, egg, onion, carrot, coconut aminos, sage, garlic powder, salt, and pepper, using your hands to ensure they are well combined.

2. Grease the slow cooker insert with your favorite Paleo fat or oil.

3. In the bottom of the slow cooker, form the meat mixture into a loaf.

4. Cover and cook on low for 8 hours, and serve.

A LITTLE LESS PALEO: To add some spicy zip to your meatloaf, add a tablespoon of sriracha to the meat mixture. Alternatively, add some hot mustard or the Orange-Chili-Garlic Sauce (page 28). Coconut aminos is basically coconut tree sap. It's a great alternative to soy sauce. Look for it in health food stores and online.

PER SERVING CALORIES: 409; PROTEIN: 37G; CARBOHYDRATES: 12G; SUGAR: 4G; FAT: 24G; FIBER: 5G; SODIUM: 569MG

Apple AND Breakfast Sausage–Stuffed Peppers

PREP TIME: 20 MINUTES / COOK TIME: 8 HOURS

SERVES 4 Stuffed peppers for breakfast? Why not! You'll get lots of fiber from the almond meal stuffing, and the sweet peppers and apples complement the sage-flavored breakfast sausage perfectly. The result is a savory breakfast that fills you up and gives you energy to go about your day.

2 cups almond meal

8 ounces breakfast sausage links, sliced

2 apples, peeled, cored, and chopped

¼ cup apple juice

2 tablespoons coconut oil, melted

2 eggs, beaten

½ teaspoon sea salt

¼ teaspoon freshly ground black pepper

4 red, yellow, or orange bell peppers, tops, ribs, and seeds removed

Water to fill the slow cooker about 1 inch

1. In a large bowl, stir well to combine the almond meal, sausage links, apples, apple juice, coconut oil, eggs, salt, and pepper.

2. Spoon the mixture into the prepared peppers.

3. Place the peppers, stuffed-side up, in the slow cooker. Add about 1 inch of water in the bottom of the slow cooker.

4. Cover and cook on low for 8 hours, and serve.

PRECOOKING: For a richer sausage flavor, sauté the sausage in the coconut oil. Stir in the almond meal, apple juice, and apples, stirring to coat the almond meal with the fat and liquids. Allow to cool completely before stirring in the eggs, salt, and pepper, and stuffing the peppers.

PER SERVING CALORIES: 649; PROTEIN: 25G; CARBOHYDRATES: 32G; SUGAR: 18G; FAT: 49G; FIBER: 11G; SODIUM: 696MG

Jalapeño, Sausage, AND Egg Casserole

PREP TIME: 10 MINUTES / COOK TIME: 8 HOURS

QP

SERVES 6 This casserole has a Mexican flare that gets your taste buds going first thing in the morning. Using canned, chopped chiles speeds up the process, as you won't have to seed and chop your own jalapeños. You can use your favorite breakfast sausage links, or make your own sausage for this casserole (see Slow Cooker Breakfast Meatloaf, page 40).

8 eggs

½ cup unsweetened almond milk

1 teaspoon chili powder

½ teaspoon ground cumin

½ teaspoon ground coriander

½ teaspoon sea salt

¼ teaspoon freshly ground black pepper

2 (4-ounce) cans chopped green chiles, drained

4 scallions, chopped

8 uncooked breakfast sausage links, sliced

Paleo-friendly fat or oil, for greasing

1 cup Cooked Salsa (page 29)

1. In a large bowl, whisk together the eggs, almond milk, chili powder, cumin, coriander, salt, and pepper.

2. Fold in the chiles, scallions, and breakfast sausage.

3. Using the Paleo-friendly fat or oil of your choice, grease the slow cooker insert.

4. Pour in the egg and sausage mixture.

5. Cover and cook on low for 8 hours.

6. Serve topped with the salsa.

A LITTLE LESS PALEO: When you fold in the sausage, peppers, and onions, also fold in ½ cup grated grass-fed Monterey Jack cheese or pepper jack cheese.

PER SERVING CALORIES: 286; PROTEIN: 16G; CARBOHYDRATES: 31G; SUGAR: 16G; FAT: 13G; FIBER: 12G; SODIUM: 681MG

Linguica AND Bell Pepper Scramble

PREP TIME: 10 MINUTES / COOK TIME: 8 HOURS

(QP)

SERVES 6 Linguica is a Portuguese sausage seasoned with garlic and paprika. It is savory, smoky, and delicious—and it imparts those flavors to this tasty scramble made with sweet bell peppers and eggs. Andouille or kielbasa will work just as well in this dish. If you can find it, use smoked paprika in the eggs to give the breakfast even more sweet smokiness.

8 eggs

¼ cup unsweetened almond milk

1 tablespoon honey

1 teaspoon ground sweet paprika or smoked paprika

½ teaspoon sea salt

¼ teaspoon freshly ground black pepper

8 ounces linguica, sliced

1 red bell pepper, seeded, stemmed, and chopped

Paleo-friendly fat or oil, for greasing

1. In a large bowl, whisk together the eggs, almond milk, honey, paprika, salt, and pepper.

2. Fold in the linguica and bell pepper.

3. Using your favorite Paleo-friendly fat or oil, grease the slow cooker insert.

4. Pour in the egg mixture.

5. Cover and cook on low for 8 hours, and serve.

NUTRITION HIGHLIGHT: Red bell peppers contain more than 100 percent of your recommended daily allowance for vitamin C. They are also a good source of vitamins A and B6.

PER SERVING CALORIES: 223; PROTEIN: 14G; CARBOHYDRATES: 6G; SUGAR: 5G; FAT: 16G; FIBER: 1G; SODIUM: 512MG

Sweet Potato AND Sausage Frittata

PREP TIME: 15 MINUTES / COOK TIME: 8 HOURS

SERVES 6 This is a pretty basic frittata, but it's really delicious. Breakfast sausage imparts flavor, while the sweet potato adds a sweet earthiness to the eggs. Finishing with a quick gremolata (a condiment classically made of lemon zest, garlic, and parsley) boosts the flavor even more, adding a bright and fresh herbal flavor to the breakfast that you'll enjoy.

8 eggs

¼ cup unsweetened almond milk

1 teaspoon sea salt, divided

½ teaspoon garlic powder

¼ teaspoon freshly ground black pepper

2 sweet potatoes, peeled and grated

4 ounces mushrooms, sliced

8 ounces breakfast sausage links, sliced

Paleo-friendly fat or oil, for greasing

½ cup chopped fresh parsley

2 garlic cloves, minced

Zest of 1 orange

1. In a small bowl, whisk together the eggs, almond milk, and ½ teaspoon of salt with the garlic powder and pepper.

2. Fold in the sweet potatoes, mushrooms, and breakfast sausage.

3. Using your favorite Paleo friendly fat or oil, grease the slow cooker insert.

4. Pour in the egg mixture. Cover and cook on low for 8 hours.

5. In a small bowl, stir together the parsley and the remaining ½ teaspoon of salt with the garlic and orange zest.

6. Sprinkle the parsley mixture over the frittata just before serving.

NUTRITION HIGHLIGHT: Parsley is a rich source of vitamin K, a fat-soluble vitamin essential for blood clotting. It's also a good source of vitamin C and iron.

PER SERVING CALORIES: 505; PROTEIN: 35G; CARBOHYDRATES: 15G; SUGAR: 1G; FAT: 33G; FIBER: 2G; SODIUM: 1,129MG

Smoked Salmon, Shiitake AND Spinach Frittata

PREP TIME: 10 MINUTES / COOK TIME: 8 HOURS

SERVES 6 The smoky flavor of the salmon complements the earthy, meaty flavor of shiitake mushrooms, while the spinach adds a pop of color and a bright vegetal flavor to this tasty frittata. If you can't find salmon that has been smoked without sugar or chemicals, you can substitute with your favorite fish or meat in its place.

10 eggs

¼ cup unsweetened almond milk

1 teaspoon garlic powder

1 teaspoon Orange-Chili-Garlic Sauce (page 28)

½ teaspoon sea salt

¼ teaspoon freshly ground black pepper

8 ounces smoked salmon, flaked

8 ounces shiitake mushrooms, sliced

2 cups baby spinach

Paleo-friendly fat or oil, for greasing

1. In a large bowl, whisk together the eggs, almond milk, garlic powder, Orange-Chili-Garlic Sauce, salt, and pepper.

2. Fold in the smoked salmon, mushrooms and spinach.

3. Using your favorite Paleo oil or fat, grease the slow cooker insert.

4. Pour in the egg mixture.

5. Cover and cook on low for 8 hours, and serve.

> **NUTRITION HIGHLIGHT:** Salmon is high in omega-3 fatty acids, which help your body fight inflammation. Spinach is an excellent source of antioxidants to help your body eliminate cell damage from oxidative stress, and shiitake mushrooms are high in the mineral selenium.

PER SERVING CALORIES: 176; PROTEIN: 17G; CARBOHYDRATES: 7G; SUGAR: 2G; FAT: 9G; FIBER: 1G; SODIUM: 1,134MG

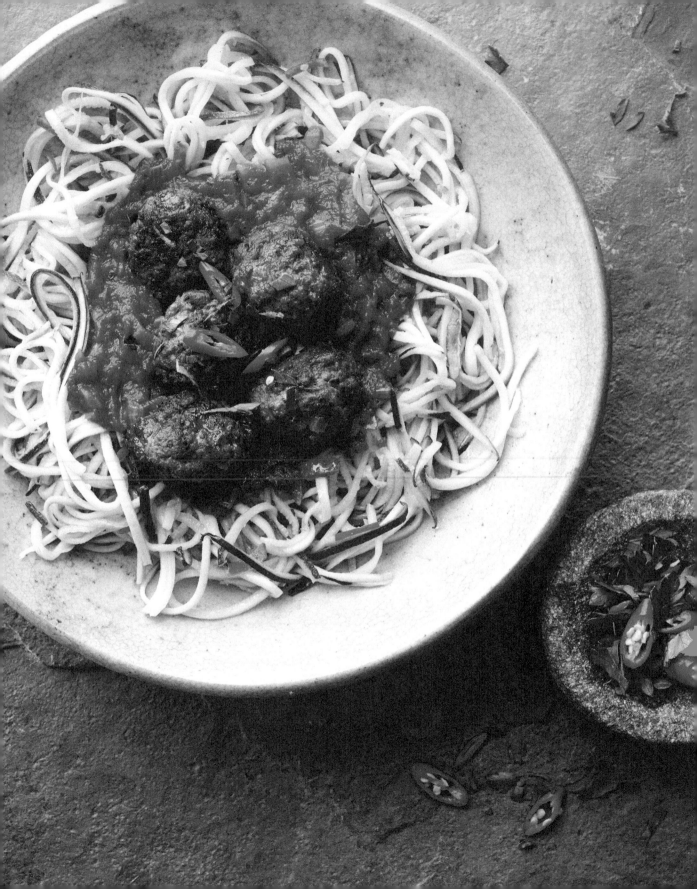

Appetizers and Sides

Caramelized Onions

PREP TIME: 10 MINUTES / COOK TIME: 9 TO 10 HOURS

SERVES 4 Caramelizing onions on the stovetop takes about 45 minutes of active time, but in a slow cooker you can add the onions and walk away. Caramelized onions add deep savory and sweet flavors to dishes. They are also delicious topping for a steak or a burger and make a tasty addition to soups and stews. They freeze well. Freeze them in half-cup servings in a tightly sealed container or zip-top bag for up to a year.

6 onions, sliced

2 tablespoons Paleo-friendly fat or oil

½ teaspoon sea salt

1. In the slow cooker, toss the onions with the fat and salt.

2. Cover and cook on low for 8 hours.

3. Remove the lid and continue to simmer for 1 to 2 hours more, until excess water has evaporated, and serve.

A LITTLE LESS PALEO: Add a buttery flavor to the onions by replacing the oil with 2 to 3 tablespoons of melted unsalted butter. You can also add a smoky flavor by replacing the oil with rendered bacon fat.

PER SERVING CALORIES: 126; PROTEIN: 2G; CARBOHYDRATES: 15G; SUGAR: 7G; FAT: 7G; FIBER: 4G; SODIUM: 241MG

Baked Sweet Potatoes

PREP TIME: 5 MINUTES / COOK TIME: 8 HOURS

LS QP

SERVES 4 Baked sweet potatoes make a delicious side dish, and they're easy to top with your favorite topping, whether it is whipped butter, salt and pepper, Cooked Salsa (page 29), Marinara Sauce (page 31), or stir-fry meat and vegetables to make them a meal. These sweet potatoes are super easy to make—you'll spend only about 5 minutes preparing them.

4 sweet potatoes

1. Prick each sweet potato several times with a fork.

2. Wrap the sweet potatoes individually in aluminum foil, and put them in the slow cooker.

3. Cover and cook on low for 8 hours, and serve.

NUTRITION HIGHLIGHT:
A medium-size sweet potato baked in the skin is nutritionally dense. It's high in vitamins B6, A, D, and C, as well as iron, potassium, and magnesium.

PER SERVING CALORIES: 100; PROTEIN: 2G; CARBOHYDRATES: 23G; SUGAR: 9G; FAT: <1G; FIBER: 4G; SODIUM: 40MG

Sweet Potato Mash

PREP TIME: 10 MINUTES / COOK TIME: 8 HOURS

SERVES 6 If you're looking for a starchy side dish with lots of flavor, mashed sweet potatoes are an excellent choice. This version adds Chinese five spice powder (a blend of star anise, cloves, cinnamon, fennel seeds, and Sichuan pepper) for extra flavor. Find it at many grocery stores, ethnic markets, and online. The spice blend perfectly complements the sweet potato, while coconut milk adds a rich creaminess to the dish. It's a delicious way to eat healthy sweet potatoes.

6 sweet potatoes, peeled and cut into 2-inch pieces

1½ cups Vegetable Stock (page 22)

¼ cup coconut milk

1½ teaspoons Chinese five spice powder

1 teaspoon sea salt

1. In the slow cooker, combine the sweet potatoes and vegetable stock.

2. Cover and cook on low for 8 hours.

3. Add the coconut milk, Chinese five spice powder, and salt.

4. Using a potato masher, mash the sweet potatoes until smooth, or purée in a blender or food processor, and serve.

> **A LITTLE LESS PALEO:** For a rich, buttery flavor, add 2 tablespoons of butter when you add the coconut milk, salt, and Chinese five spice.

PER SERVING CALORIES: 269; PROTEIN: 3G; CARBOHYDRATES: 57G; SUGAR: 2G; FAT: 3G; FIBER: 8G; SODIUM: 522MG

Sweet AND Spicy Kale

PREP TIME: 10 MINUTES / COOK TIME: 8 HOURS

SERVES 6 Adding a little sweetness and a little spice to kale balances out some of the bitterness of this dark, leafy green, making it a really delicious side dish. When preparing the kale, trim away the large center stems, which tend to be a little on the tough side, leaving only the leaves for the dish.

¼ cup pure maple syrup

1 teaspoon garlic powder

Juice and zest of 1 orange

1 teaspoon sea salt

¼ to ½ teaspoon red pepper flakes

¼ teaspoon freshly ground black pepper

2 pounds kale, stems trimmed

1. In a small bowl, whisk together the maple syrup, garlic powder, orange juice and zest, salt, red pepper flakes, and pepper.

2. In the slow cooker, add the syrup mixture to the kale, tossing to coat.

3. Cover and cook on low for 8 hours, and serve.

NUTRITION HIGHLIGHT: Kale is considered a superfood for good reason: It's high in vitamins K, A, and C, as well as manganese, copper, and fiber.

PER SERVING CALORIES: 125; PROTEIN: 5G; CARBOHYDRATES: 29G; SUGAR: 11G; FAT: <1G; FIBER: 3G; SODIUM: 379MG

Braised Fennel AND Artichokes

PREP TIME: 10 MINUTES / COOK TIME: 8 HOURS

SERVES 6 Fennel has a savory, light licorice flavor that goes very well with the slight bitterness of the artichokes. Sun-dried tomatoes add a hint of sweetness, while herbs and spices add fresh and bright notes. This is excellent as a meal, or as a side to a meat dish. Trim away the stems and fronds from the fennel bulbs, but save them for use in Vegetable Stock (page 22) or Bone Broth (page 26).

2 fennel bulbs, sliced

2 (15-ounce) cans organic artichoke
   hearts, drained

1 red onion, sliced

1½ cups Vegetable Stock (page 22)

1 cup sun-dried tomatoes

1 teaspoon dried oregano

1 teaspoon garlic powder

½ teaspoon dried thyme

½ teaspoon sea salt

½ teaspoon freshly ground black pepper

1. In the slow cooker, combine the fennel bulbs, artichoke hearts, onion, Vegetable Stock, tomatoes, oregano, garlic powder, thyme, salt, and pepper.

2. Cover and cook on low for 8 hours, and serve.

> **A LITTLE LESS PALEO:** Adding wine bumps up the flavor. Replace ½ cup of the stock with a dry white wine, such as Chardonnay.

PER SERVING CALORIES: 116; PROTEIN: 7G; CARBOHYDRATES: 24G; SUGAR: 3G; FAT: 1G; FIBER: 11G; SODIUM: 523MG

Honey-Glazed Root Vegetables

PREP TIME: 15 MINUTES / COOK TIME: 8 HOURS

SERVES 4 These vegetables are sweet, salty, slightly acidic, savory, tender, and just a little starchy, with a hint of heat all of which makes them incredibly satisfying. One of the best things about this recipe (aside from its flavor) is its versatility. You can change up the veggies to add any root vegetables or tubers that suit your palate, or are available seasonally.

8 ounces baby carrots

1 fennel bulb, sliced

2 cups pearl onions, peeled

2 turnips, peeled and sliced

1 celeriac bulb, peeled and cut into cubes

¼ cup balsamic vinegar

¼ cup honey

Juice and zest of 1 orange

1 teaspoon garlic powder

¼ teaspoon dried red pepper flakes

1 cup rainbow chard (or any chard), chopped

1. In the slow cooker, combine the carrots, fennel bulb, onions, turnips, celeriac bulb, vinegar, honey, orange juice and zest, garlic powder, and red pepper flakes.

2. Cover and cook on low for 7½ hours.

3. Stir in the chard, turn the heat to high, and cook for 30 minutes more before serving.

> **SEASONAL INGREDIENTS:** You can vary the root vegetables you choose by season. For example, use beets and golden beets in the spring or fall, or turnips and parsnips in summer and autumn

PER SERVING CALORIES: 210; PROTEIN: 5G; CARBOHYDRATES: 51G; SUGAR: 32G; FAT: <1G; FIBER: 5G; SODIUM: 219MG

Sweet AND Sour Cabbage AND Apples

PREP TIME: 15 MINUTES / COOK TIME: 8 HOURS

SERVES 6 Cabbage and apples make a flavorful combination, and when you add the sweetness of honey, the sourness of vinegar, and a bit of heat from Orange-Chili-Garlic Sauce, you've got a dish that hits all the high notes. This is a delicious and satisfying side that has an addictive flavor.

¼ cup honey

¼ cup apple cider vinegar

2 tablespoons Orange-Chili-Garlic Sauce (page 28)

1 teaspoon sea salt

3 sweet-tart apples (such as Braeburn), peeled, cored, and sliced

2 heads green cabbage, cored and shredded

1 sweet red onion, thinly sliced

1. In a small bowl, whisk together the honey, vinegar, Orange-Chili-Garlic Sauce.

2. In the slow cooker, combine the honey mixture with the apples, cabbage, and onion.

3. Cover and cook on low for 8 hours, and serve.

NUTRITION HIGHLIGHT: Cabbage is an excellent source of fiber, with about 18 grams per small head. It's also high in vitamins K and C, so it serves as a good source of nutrients.

PER SERVING CALORIES: 164; PROTEIN: 4G; CARBOHYDRATES: 41G; SUGAR: 31G; FAT: <1G; FIBER: 9G; SODIUM: 437MG

Roasted Garlic Cauliflower Mash

PREP TIME: 10 MINUTES / COOK TIME: 8 HOURS

QP

SERVES 6 Roasted garlic adds a deep caramelized flavor to this starchy cauliflower mash, which is a flavorful replacement for mashed potatoes. Although the recipe calls for grass-fed butter, you can eliminate this if you are sensitive to dairy. Instead, replace it with an equal amount of olive oil or melted duck fat.

2 heads cauliflower, broken into florets

1½ cups Vegetable Stock (page 22)

3 tablespoons grass-fed butter, melted

1 bulb Roasted Garlic (page 33)

1 teaspoon sea salt

⅛ teaspoon freshly ground black pepper

1. In the slow cooker, combine the cauliflower and Vegetable Stock.

2. Cover and cook on low for 8 hours.

3. Add the butter and squeeze the garlic from the skins into the cauliflower. Add the salt and pepper.

4. Using a potato masher, mash the cauliflower mixture until reasonably smooth, or purée in a blender or food processor, and serve.

NUTRITION HIGHLIGHT: An entire head of cauliflower has just 146 calories, and it's extremely nutritious. The whole head has almost 5 times your recommended daily allowance for vitamin C, and it's also a rich source of vitamin B6 and magnesium.

PER SERVING CALORIES: 83; PROTEIN: 3G; CARBOHYDRATES: 5G; SUGAR: 2G; FAT: 6G; FIBER: 2G; SODIUM: 530MG

Garlic AND Herb Mushrooms

PREP TIME: 10 MINUTES / COOK TIME: 8 HOURS

(QP)

SERVES 6 The most work involved in this savory dish is cleaning the mushrooms. To do so, simply wipe them with a paper towel, and trim off a small part of the end of each stem. This dish is earthy and fragrant, with savory herbs and a deep, rich, meaty flavor from the mushrooms. While this calls for cremini mushrooms, you can also use button mushrooms, or any seasonal wild mushrooms if you wish.

¼ cup Vegetable Stock (page 22)

2 tablespoons extra-virgin olive oil

1 tablespoon Dijon mustard

1 teaspoon dried thyme

1 teaspoon sea salt

½ teaspoon dried rosemary

¼ teaspoon freshly ground black pepper

2 pounds cremini mushrooms, cleaned

6 garlic cloves, minced

¼ cup chopped fresh parsley

1. In a small bowl, whisk together the Vegetable Stock, olive oil, mustard, thyme, salt, rosemary, and pepper.

2. In the slow cooker, combine the mushrooms and garlic with the stock mixture.

3. Cover and cook on low for 8 hours.

4. Stir in the parsley before serving.

A LITTLE LESS PALEO: Dry red wine complements the earthy flavor of the mushrooms perfectly. Try replacing the stock with a big, dry red wine, such as Pinot Noir or Grenache.

PER SERVING CALORIES: 92; PROTEIN: 4G; CARBOHYDRATES: 8G; SUGAR: 3G; FAT: 5G; FIBER: 1G; SODIUM: 353MG

Garlic Chicken Livers

PREP TIME: 10 MINUTES / COOK TIME: 8 HOURS

SERVES 6 Organ meats are healthy Paleo foods, and chicken livers make a wonderful snack, appetizer, or side. These livers are cooked with smoky bacon that takes away some of the gaminess, mushrooms that add earthy flavor, and garlic and herbs for freshness and zip. You can leave the livers whole and eat them as a snack, or you can purée the entire recipe in a food processor or blender to make a paté you can spread on vegetables.

1 pound chicken livers

8 garlic cloves, minced

8 ounces cremini mushrooms, quartered

4 slices uncooked bacon, chopped

1 onion, chopped

1 cup Bone Broth (page 26)

1 teaspoon dried thyme

1 teaspoon dried rosemary

1 teaspoon sea salt

1 teaspoon freshly ground black pepper

¼ cup chopped fresh parsley

1. In the slow cooker, combine the livers, garlic, mushrooms, bacon, onion, Bone Broth, thyme, rosemary, salt, and pepper.

2. Cover and cook on low for 8 hours.

3. Stir in the parsley before serving.

> **A LITTLE LESS PALEO:** Add a rich wine flavor to the livers. To do this, replace the broth with a dry white wine such as Chardonnay.

PER SERVING CALORIES: 210; PROTEIN: 24G; CARBOHYDRATES: 6G; SUGAR: 2G; FAT: 9G; FIBER: 1G; SODIUM: 720MG

Kung Pao Chicken Legs

PREP TIME: 10 MINUTES / COOK TIME: 8 HOURS

SERVES 8 Kung pao chicken is a spicy Asian chicken that is juicy and flavorful. Coating chicken drumsticks with kung pao sauce makes this finger food sticky but delicious. While traditional kung pao chicken has peanuts, this recipe uses shelled pistachios, which add tasty crunch to the moist chicken. Extracted from fish fermented with sea salt, Asian fish sauce is used as a condiment in South Asian cuisines. You can find it in well-stocked supermarkets, ethnic markets, and online.

2 tablespoons coconut aminos

2 tablespoons Orange-Chili-Garlic Sauce (page 28)

2 tablespoons pure maple syrup

Juice of 1 orange

2 tablespoons arrowroot powder

1 tablespoon apple cider vinegar

1 tablespoon Asian fish sauce

8 chicken drumsticks

1 cup shelled pistachios

4 scallions, sliced on an angle

1. In a small bowl, whisk together the coconut aminos, Orange-Chili-Garlic Sauce, maple syrup, orange juice, arrowroot powder, apple cider vinegar, and fish sauce.

2. Toss the sauce mixture with the drumsticks, pistachios, and scallions, and add to the slow cooker.

3. Cover and cook on low for 8 hours, and serve.

SEASONAL INGREDIENTS: When chile peppers are in season, add 1 or 2 thinly sliced chiles to the mixture before putting it in the slow cooker. It will bump up the heat a bit, and add tremendous flavor.

PER SERVING CALORIES: 206; PROTEIN: 16G; CARBOHYDRATES: 14G; SUGAR: 6G; FAT: 10G; FIBER: 2G; SODIUM: 243MG

Honey Jalapeño-Glazed Chicken Wings

PREP TIME: 10 MINUTES / COOK TIME: 8 HOURS

SERVES 8 Sweet, spicy, and salty flavors make these savory chicken wings addictive. They're the perfect game-day snack; nobody will even suspect they are a healthy Paleo appetizer. For a little added heat, feel free to leave a few of the jalapeño seeds in the mix, or remove all the seeds to tone it down a bit.

¼ cup honey

Juice and zest of 1 lime

3 jalapeño peppers, minced

2 tablespoons coconut aminos

1 teaspoon garlic powder

¼ teaspoon freshly ground black pepper

3 pounds chicken wings, separated into drumettes and wing sections

1. In a small bowl, whisk together the honey, lime juice and zest, jalapeños, coconut aminos, garlic powder, and pepper.

2. In the slow cooker, toss the honey mixture together with the chicken wings.

3. Cover and cook on low for 8 hours, and serve.

NUTRITION HIGHLIGHT: Chile peppers like jalapeños contain capsaicin. Capsaicin has anti-inflammatory and vasodilation properties that can promote healthy blood flow.

PER SERVING CALORIES: 365; PROTEIN: 49G; CARBOHYDRATES: 11G; SUGAR: 9G; FAT: 13G; FIBER: 0G; SODIUM: 151MG

Jalapeño Poppers

PREP TIME: 20 MINUTES / COOK TIME: 8 HOURS

SERVES 8 These little bites of heaven are spicy and savory. They make great appetizers, and they're perfect for a party where you want to make sure there's something Paleo there for you to eat. Smoky bacon sets off the heat of the jalapeños. Remember to remove all the seeds from the peppers to tone down the heat just a bit.

16 jalapeño peppers, halved lengthwise, seeds, stems, and ribs removed

½ pound bulk chorizo

16 thin-cut bacon slices, cut in half

1. Fill each pepper half with chorizo and wrap in a slice of bacon, securing with a toothpick.

2. Set the poppers in the slow cooker cut-side up.

3. Cover and cook on low for 8 hours, and serve.

A LITTLE LESS PALEO: With chorizo and jalapeños, these poppers have a little bit of heat. Cool them down by mixing ½ cup of grated Cheddar cheese with the chorizo and serving some grass-fed sour cream on the side as a dip.

PER SERVING CALORIES: 387; PROTEIN: 26G; CARBOHYDRATES: 3G; SUGAR: 1G; FAT: 29G; FIBER: 1G; SODIUM: 2,185MG

Apple, Sausage AND Herb Dressing

PREP TIME: 20 MINUTES / COOK TIME: 8 HOURS

SERVES 6 If you like Thanksgiving dressing or stuffing, then you'll really love this Paleo version. It's flavored with sage sausage and sweet apples along with fragrant herbs. It's a really delicious replacement for the traditional grain-filled versions. Best of all, it cooks well in a slow cooker with no supervision, and your house will smell like a holiday whenever you make it.

1 pound breakfast sausage links, sliced

2 sweet-tart apples (such as Braeburn), peeled, cored, and chopped

4 cups almond meal

2 cups Vegetable Stock (page 22)

2 eggs, beaten

1 onion, chopped

1 teaspoon garlic powder

1 teaspoon dried sage

1 teaspoon dried thyme

1 teaspoon sea salt

¼ teaspoon freshly ground black pepper

1. In the slow cooker, combine the sausage, apples, almond meal, Vegetable Stock, eggs, onion, garlic powder, sage, thyme, salt, and pepper.

2. Cover and cook on low for 8 hours, and serve.

PRECOOKING: To add a depth of flavor, brown the onions and sausage in 2 tablespoons of fat or oil before adding to the slow cooker.

PER SERVING CALORIES: 403; PROTEIN: 21G; CARBOHYDRATES: 22G; SUGAR: 9G; FAT: 28G; FIBER: 8G; SODIUM: 937MG

Caramelized Onion Meatballs

PREP TIME: 20 MINUTES / COOK TIME: 8 HOURS

SERVES 8 If you're looking for a satisfying, savory bite, you can't go wrong with these meatballs, which make a delicious appetizer, snack, or main course. The meatballs freeze very well, storing up to 1 year in zip-top bags. They are also delicious added to soups, or as a filling for lettuce wraps.

1 pound ground beef

1 pound ground pork

1 cup Caramelized Onions (page 48)

1 cup almond meal

1 egg, beaten

1 teaspoon dried thyme

1 teaspoon garlic powder

1 teaspoon Dijon mustard

1 teaspoon sea salt

¼ teaspoon freshly ground black pepper

1. In a large bowl, mix together the beef, pork, Caramelized Onions, almond meal, egg, thyme, garlic powder, mustard, salt, and pepper.

2. Form into 1-inch meatballs, and place in the slow cooker.

3. Cover and cook on low for 8 hours, and serve.

PRECOOKING: To add even more flavor, brown the meatballs in 2 tablespoons of fat or oil before adding them to the slow cooker. Doing so will add deep, savory flavors to the dish.

PER SERVING CALORIES: 277; PROTEIN: 36G; CARBOHYDRATES: 6G; SUGAR: 2G; FAT: 12G; FIBER: 2G; SODIUM: 320MG

Italian Meatballs Marinara

PREP TIME: 20 MINUTES / COOK TIME: 8 HOURS

SERVES 8 While these savory, garlicky Italian meatballs make a great appetizer, they're also a terrific topper for zucchini "noodles," and they're delicious as a filling for a lettuce wrap. Make the Marinara Sauce ahead of time, freeze a batch, and then thaw it to make these tasty meatballs.

1 pound bulk Italian sausage

1 pound ground beef

1 teaspoon garlic powder

1 teaspoon Italian seasoning

2 cups Marinara Sauce (page 31)

2 tablespoons extra-virgin olive oil

3 medium zucchini, cut into noodles using a veggie peeler or spiralizer

1. In a large bowl, mix the sausage, ground beef, garlic powder, and Italian seasoning.

2. Roll into 1-inch meatballs and place in the slow cooker.

3. Pour in the Marinara Sauce.

4. Cover and cook on low for 8 hours.

5. In a large sauté pan over medium-high heat, heat the olive oil until it shimmers. Add the zucchini noodles and cook, stirring occasionally, for 5 minutes.

6. Serve the zucchini topped with the meatballs and sauce.

A LITTLE LESS PALEO: For a cheesy flavor, add ½ cup of grated Parmesan cheese to the meatballs.

PER SERVING CALORIES: 355; PROTEIN: 29G; CARBOHYDRATES: 9G; SUGAR: 6G; FAT: 22G; FIBER: 2G; SODIUM: 719MG

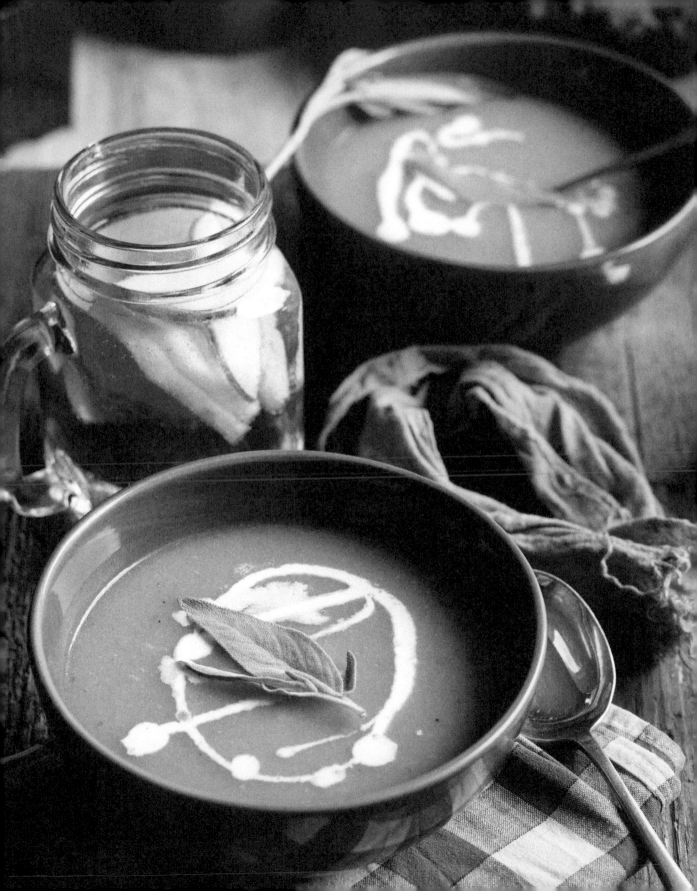

Soups and Stews

Italian Balsamic-Onion Soup

PREP TIME: 15 MINUTES / COOK TIME: 8 HOURS

SERVES 6 Similar to French onion soup, this savory soup gets a hint of sweetness from the balsamic vinegar and slow cooked onions. The soup is warming and hearty, perfect for a fall or winter dinner or lunch. It freezes well, so you can make a big batch and store it in single-serving containers for up to a year for meals on the go.

5 red onions, thinly sliced

8 cups Bone Broth (page 26) made with beef bones

¼ cup balsamic vinegar

1 teaspoon garlic powder

1 teaspoon dried thyme

1 teaspoon sea salt

¼ teaspoon freshly ground black pepper

1. In the slow cooker, combine the onions, Bone Broth, vinegar, garlic powder, thyme, salt, and pepper.

2. Cover and cook on low for 8 hours, and serve.

A LITTLE LESS PALEO: If you're looking to duplicate the French onion soup experience, add ¼ cup of grated Gruyère cheese to each bowl right before serving.

PER SERVING CALORIES: 92; PROTEIN: 8G; CARBOHYDRATES: 11G; SUGAR: 5G; FAT: 2G; FIBER: 2G; SODIUM: 1,334MG

Sweet Potato AND Leek Soup

PREP TIME: 10 MINUTES / COOK TIME: 8 HOURS

SERVES 6 Sweet potatoes and leeks are a great combination. The leeks add a savory, oniony bite, while the sweet potatoes add earthy richness to this simple soup. It's also really quick to make, coming together in less than 10 minutes, making it a perfect meal for busy days. You don't have to purée the soup at the end if you don't want to—it will just be a bit chunkier.

6 cups peeled and cubed sweet potatoes

2 leeks (whites and greens), sliced

6 cups Vegetable Stock (page 22)

1 teaspoon dried thyme

1 teaspoon sea salt

¼ teaspoon freshly ground black pepper

1. In the slow cooker, combine the sweet potatoes, leeks, Vegetable Stock, thyme, salt, and pepper.

2. Cover and cook on low for 8 hours.

3. If you wish, mash the potatoes with a potato masher or purée the soup in a food processor, blender, or using an immersion blender before serving.

A LITTLE LESS PALEO: To give this soup richness and body, add some cream. Just before serving and after puréeing (if you choose), stir in 1 cup of heavy cream.

PER SERVING CALORIES: 234; PROTEIN: 8G; CARBOHYDRATES: 47G; SUGAR: 3G; FAT: 2G; FIBER: 8G; SODIUM: 1,095MG

Butternut Squash and Pear Soup

PREP TIME: 10 MINUTES / COOK TIME: 8 HOURS

QP

SERVES 6 This quick soup is a combination of sweet and savory. Pears add a mellow sweetness to rich butternut squash, while onions, garlic, and herbs add savory notes. You can freeze this soup for meals on the go, so make up a double or triple batch if you like, and store it tightly sealed in your freezer for up to a year.

6 cups butternut squash, peeled, seeded, and cut into cubes

3 pears, peeled, cored, and chopped

6 cups Vegetable Stock (page 22)

1 onion, chopped

1 teaspoon garlic powder

1 teaspoon dried rosemary

1 teaspoon sea salt

¼ teaspoon freshly ground black pepper

1 cup coconut milk

Fresh sage leaves (optional)

1. In the slow cooker, combine the butternut squash, pears, Vegetable Stock, onion, garlic powder, rosemary, salt, and pepper.

2. Cover and cook on low for 8 hours.

3. In a blender or food processor, or using an immersion blender, purée the soup.

4. Stir in the coconut milk. If you'd like, reserve ¼ cup to drizzle on top just before serving.

5. Top with fresh sage leaves (if using), and serve.

NUTRITION HIGHLIGHT: Pears are high in fiber, copper, and vitamin C. They also contain vitamin K and are relatively low in calories, with about 100 calories per medium pear.

PER SERVING CALORIES: 264; PROTEIN: 8G; CARBOHYDRATES: 38G; SUGAR: 16G; FAT: 11G; FIBER: 8G; SODIUM: 1,089MG

Pumpkin-Curry Soup

PREP TIME: 10 MINUTES / COOK TIME: 8 HOURS

SERVES 6 Canned pumpkin makes this soup come together very quickly. Make sure you buy pure pumpkin, and not pumpkin pie mix, which has added flavors. This fragrant soup smells delicious as it cooks, with scents of ginger, curry, and garam masala, an Indian spice blend available in supermarkets and ethnic markets. Coconut milk adds luscious richness and creaminess, turning it into a hearty meal.

2 (29-ounce) cans pumpkin purée

1 onion, chopped

5 cups Vegetable Stock (page 22)

1 teaspoon garlic powder

1 teaspoon garam masala

1 teaspoon curry powder

1 teaspoon sea salt

½ teaspoon ground ginger

2 tablespoons chopped fresh cilantro

1 cup coconut milk

1. In the slow cooker, stir to combine the pumpkin, onion, Vegetable Stock, garlic powder, garam masala, curry powder, salt, and ginger.

2. Cover and cook on low for 8 hours.

3. Stir in the cilantro and coconut milk just before serving.

> **NUTRITION HIGHLIGHT:** Pumpkin is a type of winter squash, in the same family as butternut squash, and it's high in nutritional value. It contains vitamins A and C, along with vitamin B6, copper, and manganese. It's also high in fiber.

PER SERVING CALORIES: 228; PROTEIN: 8G; CARBOHYDRATES: 28G; SUGAR: 12G; FAT: 12G; FIBER: 9G; SODIUM: 970MG

Spicy Coconut AND Shrimp Chowder

PREP TIME: 20 MINUTES / COOK TIME: 8½ HOURS

SERVES 6 This spicy chowder is a treat for your taste buds, with sweet and briny shrimp, creamy coconut, and hot chile peppers. It's a hearty soup that freezes well and makes an excellent meal on the go. To save time, purchase precooked baby shrimp (wild caught) and stir them in at the very end of cooking. That will keep the shrimp tender and flavorful.

6 cups Fish Stock (page 24)

2 tablespoons arrowroot powder

½ cup chopped chile peppers (of your choice—jalapeños, Anaheim, etc)

2 cups peeled and cubed sweet potatoes

1 onion, chopped

2 carrots, peeled and chopped

1 teaspoon garlic powder

1 teaspoon sea salt

½ teaspoon ground ginger

Zest of 1 lime

Juice of 1 lime

1 cup coconut milk

1 pound cooked baby shrimp

¼ cup chopped fresh cilantro

1. In a large bowl, whisk together the Fish Stock and arrowroot powder.

2. Add the stock mixture to the slow cooker along with the chiles, sweet potatoes, onion, carrots, garlic powder, salt, ginger, and lime zest.

3. Cover and cook on low for 8 hours.

4. Stir in the lime juice, coconut milk, shrimp, and cilantro.

5. Cover and cook for an additional 30 minutes, and serve.

NUTRITION HIGHLIGHT: Shrimp is an excellent protein source, containing fewer than 100 calories per serving with 24 grams of protein. It's also a pretty good source of calcium and magnesium.

PER SERVING CALORIES: 293; PROTEIN: 21G; CARBOHYDRATES: 28G; SUGAR: 6G; FAT: 12G; FIBER: 5G; SODIUM: 1,235MG

Cioppino (Seafood Soup)

PREP TIME: 20 MINUTES / COOK TIME: 8½ HOURS

SERVES 6 Despite the Italian name, cioppino originated in San Francisco, and is considered an Italian American dish. The seafood soup is loaded with flavor and fragrant with Italian herbs and sweet tomato broth. Stir in the seafood during the last half hour of cooking, turning the temperature up to high so the seafood cooks through. Adding the seafood at the end keeps it moist and tender.

1 (14-ounce) can tomato sauce

7 cups Fish Stock (page 24)

1 onion, chopped

1 tablespoon Italian seasoning

1 teaspoon garlic powder

1 teaspoon sea salt

¼ teaspoon freshly ground black pepper

Pinch red pepper flakes

8 ounces cod or halibut fillets, skin removed, cut into 1-inch pieces

8 ounces shrimp, peeled and deveined

8 ounces mussels, cleaned and debearded

¼ cup chopped fresh parsley

Zest of 1 lemon

1. In the slow cooker, combine the tomato sauce, Fish Stock, onion, Italian seasoning, garlic powder, salt, pepper, and red pepper flakes.

2. Cover and cook on low for 8 hours.

3. Stir in the fish, shrimp, mussels, parsley, and lemon zest, and turn the slow cooker up to high.

4. Cover and cook for an additional 30 minutes, or until the fish is cooked through, and serve.

NUTRITION HIGHLIGHT: Fish is high in omega-3 fatty acids, which can help your body fight inflammation.

PER SERVING CALORIES: 197; PROTEIN: 29G; CARBOHYDRATES: 8G; SUGAR: 4G; FAT: 5G; FIBER: 2G; SODIUM: 1,316MG

Chicken Noodle Soup

PREP TIME: 20 MINUTES / COOK TIME: 8½ HOURS

SERVES 6 If you're craving classic comfort food, this is the recipe for you. Here, zucchini strips replace the noodles. To make them, use a vegetable peeler to cut the zucchini into long ribbons. Alternatively, if you have a spiralizer, use it to turn the zucchini into spaghetti-like noodles.

8 cups Bone Broth (page 26) made with chicken bones

1 pound boneless, skinless chicken breasts, cut into ½-inch pieces

2 carrots, peeled and sliced

2 celery stalks, chopped

1 onion, chopped

1 teaspoon garlic powder

1 teaspoon dried thyme

1 teaspoon sea salt

¼ teaspoon freshly ground black pepper

2 zucchini, cut into noodles

1. In the slow cooker, combine the Bone Broth, chicken, carrots, celery, onion, garlic powder, thyme, salt, and pepper.

2. Cover and cook on low for 8 hours.

3. Stir in the zucchini noodles, and turn the slow cooker up to high.

4. Cover and cook for an additional 30 minutes, and serve.

A LITTLE LESS PALEO: If you really want noodles, try shirataki noodles, which are made from konjac, a tuber also known as elephant yam. When you're really craving noodles, they're a great substitute for wheat noodles. They don't have a lot of flavor on their own, but they soak up the flavor of whatever you cook them in. Shop for them online and in health food stores.

PER SERVING CALORIES: 205; PROTEIN: 32G; CARBOHYDRATES: 8G; SUGAR: 4G; FAT: 5G; FIBER: 2G; SODIUM: 1,443MG

Minestrone with Italian Sausage

PREP TIME: 20 MINUTES / COOK TIME: 8 HOURS

SERVES 6 Minestrone is the perfect "dump" soup, in that you can dump ingredients of your choosing and still have it come out tasting really good. This version bumps up the flavor with Italian sausage and Italian herbs, but play with the ingredients as you like. It is a soup that freezes well, so it's an excellent choice for making a large batch for meals on the go.

1 pound Italian sausage, sliced

8 cups Bone Broth (page 26) made with beef bones

1 onion, chopped

2 zucchini, chopped

1 cup green beans, chopped

2 carrots, peeled and chopped

2 celery stalks, chopped

1 (28-ounce) can chopped tomatoes, undrained

1 teaspoon garlic powder

1 teaspoon Italian seasoning

1 teaspoon sea salt

¼ teaspoon freshly ground black pepper

Pinch red pepper flakes

1. In the slow cooker, combine the sausage, Bone Broth, onion, zucchini, green beans, carrots, celery, tomatoes and their juice, garlic powder, Italian seasoning, salt, pepper, and red pepper flakes.

2. Cover and cook on low for 8 hours.

PRECOOKING: To add a deeper flavor, brown the sausage and onions in 2 tablespoons of fat or oil before adding them to the soup. You can also make this dish a little less Paleo by substituting 1 cup of dry red wine for 1 cup of the broth.

PER SERVING CALORIES: 374; PROTEIN: 24G; CARBOHYDRATES: 16G; SUGAR: 8G; FAT: 24G; FIBER: 5G; SODIUM: 1,931MG

Chicken Vegetable Soup
WITH Asian Meatballs

PREP TIME: 20 MINUTES / COOK TIME: 8 HOURS

SERVES 6 Asian flavors of ginger, garlic, and citrus make this soup both tasty and fragrant. You don't have to stick with the veggies recommended here—try your own vegetable combinations based on what's available at the local farmers' market this week. This soup freezes well. You can either freeze the soup with the meatballs in it, or freeze the meatballs separately.

1 pound ground pork

2 tablespoons grated fresh ginger, divided

8 garlic cloves, minced, divided

1 tablespoon Orange-Chili-Garlic Sauce (page 28)

1 teaspoon Asian fish sauce

2 teaspoons sea salt, divided

8 scallions, sliced thinly on an angle, divided

4 tablespoons chopped fresh cilantro, divided

8 cups Bone Broth (page 26) made with chicken bones

1 onion, chopped

2 tablespoons coconut aminos

2 carrots, peeled and sliced

2 cups shredded cabbage

8 ounces shiitake mushrooms, sliced

¼ teaspoon freshly ground black pepper

1. In a large bowl, stir to combine the pork, 1 tablespoon of ginger, 4 garlic cloves, the Orange-Chili-Garlic Sauce, the fish sauce, 1 teaspoon of salt, 4 scallions, and 2 tablespoons of cilantro. Mix well and form into 1-inch meatballs.

2. In the slow cooker, combine the meatballs, the remaining 1 tablespoon of ginger, the remaining 4 garlic cloves, the remaining 1 teaspoon of salt, and the remaining 4 scallions with the Bone Broth, onion, coconut aminos, carrots, cabbage, mushrooms, and pepper.

3. Cover and cook on low for 8 hours.

4. Stir in the remaining 2 tablespoons of cilantro just before serving.

SEASONAL INGREDIENTS: In the fall, replace the cabbage with kale, which makes a hearty addition to this soup.

PER SERVING CALORIES: 223; PROTEIN: 28G; CARBOHYDRATES: 16G; SUGAR: 5G; FAT: 5G; FIBER: 3G; SODIUM: 1,894MG

Avgolemono Soup
WITH Lamb Meatballs

PREP TIME: 20 MINUTES / COOK TIME: 8 HOURS

SERVES 6 Avgolemono is a Greek egg and lemon sauce that adds brightness to dishes. Here it's incorporated into a soup with fragrant and savory lamb meatballs. The eggs in the sauce add a richness to the soup that is simply delicious. With unique flavor profiles, it's sure to become a family favorite. To prepare the onion for the meatballs, grate it and then wrap it in a towel and squeeze out as much water as you can.

1 pound ground lamb

1 teaspoon ground coriander

1 teaspoon ground cumin

1 onion, grated

1 teaspoon dried rosemary

1 teaspoon dried oregano

2 teaspoons sea salt, divided

½ teaspoon freshly ground black pepper, divided

6 garlic cloves, minced

8 cups Bone Broth (page 26) made with chicken bones

3 carrots, peeled and chopped

1 onion, chopped

1 teaspoon garlic powder

½ cup freshly squeezed lemon juice

2 eggs

1. In a large bowl, mix to combine the ground lamb, coriander, cumin, onion, rosemary, oregano, 1 teaspoon of salt, ¼ teaspoon of pepper, and the garlic.

2. Roll the mixture into 1-inch meatballs, and place them in the slow cooker.

3. Add the Bone Broth, carrots, onion, garlic powder, remaining 1 teaspoon of salt, and remaining ¼ teaspoon of pepper.

4. Cover and cook on low for 8 hours.

5. In a small bowl, whisk together the lemon juice and eggs.

6. Whisk 1 tablespoon of the hot liquid from the slow cooker into the lemon and egg mixture. When it is incorporated, add 1 more tablespoon and whisk again. Repeat until you have added 4 tablespoons.

7. Pour the egg mixture in a thin stream back into the slow cooker, stirring constantly. Serve immediately.

NUTRITION HIGHLIGHT: Lemon juice does more than add bright acidity to this dish. It also has a healthy dose of antioxidants, because lemons are high in vitamin C.

PER SERVING CALORIES: 250; PROTEIN: 36G; CARBOHYDRATES: 9G; SUGAR: 4G; FAT: 7G; FIBER: 2G; SODIUM: 857MG

Caramelized Onion, Italian Sausage AND Fennel Soup

PREP TIME: 20 MINUTES / COOK TIME: 8 HOURS

SERVES 6 The caramelized onions and Italian sausage give this soup deep flavors, while the fennel adds a hint of freshness and a light anise flavor that matches the dried fennel in the Italian sausage. This soup freezes well, and you can make the Caramelized Onions ahead of time freeze them, and then thaw them before use.

8 cups Bone Broth (page 26)

1 cup Caramelized Onions (page 48)

1 fennel bulb, sliced

2 tablespoons chopped fennel fronds

8 ounces cremini mushrooms, sliced

1 pound Italian sausage, sliced

1 teaspoon garlic powder

1 teaspoon sea salt

¼ teaspoon freshly ground black pepper

Pinch red pepper flakes

1. In the slow cooker, combine the Bone Broth, Caramelized Onion, fennel bulb and fronds, mushrooms, sausage, garlic powder, salt, pepper, and red pepper flakes.

2. Cover and cook on low for 8 hours, and serve.

A LITTLE LESS PALEO: Sherry adds a rich flavor to this soup. To add it, replace 1 cup of the Bone Broth with a cup of dry sherry.

PER SERVING CALORIES: 323; PROTEIN: 19G; CARBOHYDRATES: 11G; SUGAR: 4G; FAT: 22G; FIBER: 2G; SODIUM: 1,089MG

Chicken AND Jalapeño Stew

PREP TIME: 10 MINUTES / COOK TIME: 8 HOURS

SERVES 6 Chile peppers, cilantro, and onions give this rich Mexican stew plenty of flavor and fragrance. Serve it topped with the Cooked Salsa on page 29 as well as sliced avocados, or some homemade guacamole. The stew freezes well, so it's good for big batches.

1½ pounds boneless and skinless chicken thigh meat, cut into 1-inch pieces

2 ounces bacon, chopped

2 (6-ounce) cans chopped chile peppers, undrained

8 ounces button mushrooms, halved

1 (16-ounce) can chopped tomatoes, undrained

1 onion, chopped

3 carrots, peeled and chopped

1 cup Bone Broth (page 26) made with chicken bones

1 teaspoon garlic powder

1 teaspoon dried oregano

1 teaspoon sea salt

Dash cayenne pepper

2 tablespoon chopped fresh cilantro

1. In the slow cooker, combine the chicken, bacon, chiles and their juice, mushrooms, tomatoes and their juice, onion, carrots, Bone Broth, garlic powder, oregano, salt, and pepper.

2. Cover and cook on low for 8 hours.

3. Stir in the cilantro just before serving.

A LITTLE LESS PALEO: To add a little cheesy goodness to this spicy stew, sprinkle in 1 cup of grated pepper jack cheese in the last 30 minutes of cooking. Cover the slow cooker and finish cooking, allowing the cheese to melt. Serve topped with a dollop of sour cream.

PER SERVING CALORIES: 320; PROTEIN: 40G; CARBOHYDRATES: 10G; SUGAR: 6G; FAT: 13G; FIBER: 3G; SODIUM: 783MG

Pork Chili Colorado

PREP TIME: 10 MINUTES / COOK TIME: 8 HOURS

SERVES 8 This chili is hearty and rich, with mellow spices and just a hint of heat. It's also very easy to make, coming together in about 10 minutes total. Pork shoulder is an extremely economical cut that takes well to the slow cooker. You can also make this dish with ground beef, cubed chuck steak, or chicken thighs, so the recipe is very versatile. If you use a leaner meat, add about a cup of broth to help keep it moist.

3 pounds pork shoulder, cut into 1-inch cubes

1 teaspoon garlic powder

1 onion, chopped

1 teaspoon chipotle chili powder

1 tablespoon chili powder

1 teaspoon sea salt

1. In the slow cooker, combine the pork, garlic powder, onion, chili powders, and salt.

2. Cover and cook on low for 8 hours, and serve.

SEASONAL INGREDIENTS: You can add vegetables to this, depending on what's in season. The fat, as it renders from the pork, will keep the veggies moist. Consider adding carrots, green beans, or other garden favorites.

PER SERVING CALORIES: 506; PROTEIN: 40G; CARBOHYDRATES: 2G; SUGAR: 1G; FAT: 37G; FIBER: 1G; SODIUM: 360MG

Chili Verde

PREP TIME: 20 MINUTES / COOK TIME: 8 HOURS

SERVES 6 This green chili is spicy with peppers, and has tangy tomatillos to add a bit of acidity. Find them in the produce section—they look like small green tomatoes with a papery skin. The skin should not be dried and shriveled. Just pull it off with your hands before using. Small tomatillos are sweeter. Stirring in fresh herbs at the end adds freshness that brightens the flavors of the rich stew. While the recipe calls for pork shoulder, you can replace it with any fatty meat or poultry of your choice. It freezes well.

2 pounds pork shoulder, cut into 1-inch cubes

1 cup Bone Broth (page 26)

1 onion, chopped

½ cup chopped green chiles (your choice—jalapeños, Anaheim, etc.)

6 tomatillos, chopped

1 teaspoon garlic powder

1 teaspoon ground cumin

1 teaspoon ground coriander

1 teaspoon sea salt

Juice of 1 lime

¼ cup chopped fresh cilantro

1. In the slow cooker, combine the pork, Bone Broth, onion, chiles, tomatillos, garlic powder, cumin, coriander, and salt

2. Cover and cook on low for 8 hours.

3. Stir in the lime juice and cilantro, and serve.

> **NUTRITION HIGHLIGHT:** Tomatillos are high in niacin, potassium, vitamin K, and antioxidants, making them a healthy addition to this chili.

PER SERVING CALORIES: 479; PROTEIN: 37G; CARBOHYDRATES: 7G; SUGAR: 2G; FAT: 33G; FIBER: 2G; SODIUM: 623MG

Classic Beef Stew

PREP TIME: 15 MINUTES / COOK TIME: 8 HOURS

SERVES 8 An American classic, beef stew is rich and hearty with a thick gravy and fragrant herbs. This stew makes no compromises. It is a stick-to-your-ribs meal that you can customize depending on your favorite vegetables. It is thickened with arrowroot, which is a good Paleo substitution for wheat flour or cornstarch. This makes a big batch, but it freezes well.

4 cups Bone Broth (page 26) made with beef bones

2 tablespoons arrowroot powder

1 tablespoon Dijon mustard

3 pounds beef chuck, cut into 1-inch cubes

2 ounces bacon, chopped

1 pound pearl onions, peeled

3 carrots, peeled and chopped

1 celeriac bulb, peeled and chopped

8 ounces cremini mushrooms, halved

1 teaspoon dried rosemary

1 teaspoon garlic powder

1 teaspoon dried thyme

1 teaspoon sea salt

¼ teaspoon freshly ground black pepper

¼ cup chopped fresh parsley

1. In a medium bowl, whisk together the Bone Broth, arrowroot, and mustard.

2. Add the broth mixture to the slow cooker with the beef, bacon, onions, carrots, celeriac, mushrooms, rosemary, garlic powder, thyme, salt, and pepper.

3. Cover and cook on low for 8 hours.

4. Stir in the parsley just before serving.

A LITTLE LESS PALEO: Red wine deepens the flavors of beef stew, and peas are a common addition. Replace 1 cup of the broth with 1 cup of red wine, and add 1 cup of frozen or fresh peas before cooking.

PER SERVING CALORIES: 447; PROTEIN: 59G; CARBOHYDRATES: 19G; SUGAR: 6G; FAT: 14G; FIBER: 4G; SODIUM: 698MG

Moroccan Lamb Stew

PREP TIME: 20 MINUTES / COOK TIME: 8 HOURS

SERVES 8 This stew has exotic flavors that blend together to make a fragrant, tasty dish. The lamb is juicy and tender, and the scents of the spices and citrus will fill your home. Like all good stews, this one gets even better on the second or third day, after the flavors have had time to blend.

Juice of 1 orange

2 tablespoons arrowroot powder

Zest of 1 orange

2 pounds boneless leg of lamb, cut into 1-inch pieces

2 onions, chopped

2 carrots, peeled and chopped

1 (14-ounce) can crushed tomatoes, undrained

1 cup chopped dried dates

1 teaspoon garlic powder

1 teaspoon ground ginger

1 teaspoon ground cumin

1 teaspoon sea salt

¼ teaspoon freshly ground black pepper

¼ cup chopped fresh parsley

1. In a small bowl, whisk together the orange juice and arrowroot powder.

2. Add the juice mixture to the slow cooker with the orange zest, lamb, onions, carrots, tomatoes and their juice, dates, garlic powder, ginger, cumin, salt, and pepper.

3. Cover and cook on low for 8 hours.

4. Stir in the parsley just before serving.

> **PRECOOKING:** Add deeper flavor by browning the lamb cubes before adding them to the stew. Heat 2 tablespoons of fat or oil in a sauté pan. Working in batches, brown the lamb for about 4 minutes per side.

PER SERVING CALORIES: 445; PROTEIN: 46G; CARBOHYDRATES: 40G; SUGAR: 29G; FAT: 11G; FIBER: 7G; SODIUM: 572MG

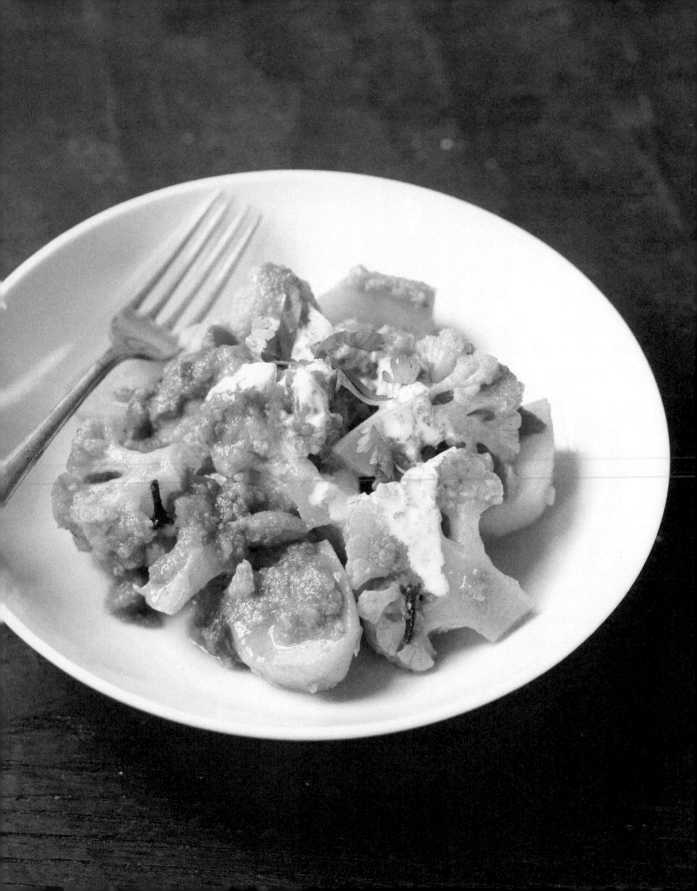

Maple-Glazed Carrots

PREP TIME: 10 MINUTES / COOK TIME: 8 HOURS

SERVES 6 Using packaged baby carrots makes this recipe a snap. Choose pure maple syrup, not the maple-flavored pancake syrup you find in the pancake aisle. While pure maple syrup is more expensive than the sugar-based, artificially flavored syrups, it makes up for the higher price in pure flavor.

¼ cup pure maple syrup

½ teaspoon ground ginger

¼ teaspoon ground nutmeg

½ teaspoon sea salt

Juice of 1 orange

1 pound baby carrots

1. In a small bowl, whisk together the syrup, ginger, nutmeg, salt, and orange juice.

2. Put the carrots in the slow cooker, and toss them with the syrup mixture.

3. Cover and cook on low for 8 hours, and serve.

NUTRITION HIGHLIGHT: Pure maple syrup is made from boiling the sap of maple trees. While it is high in sugar, it is also high in several antioxidants, according to Authority Nutrition, which notes that one study found 24 different antioxidants in pure maple syrup. While you want to limit your sugar intake, maple syrup is an excellent option for a little bit of sweetness.

PER SERVING CALORIES: 76; PROTEIN: 1G; CARBOHYDRATES: 19G; SUGAR: 14G; FAT: <1G; FIBER: 3G; SODIUM: 216MG

German-Style Celeriac

PREP TIME: 20 MINUTES / COOK TIME: 8 HOURS

SERVES 6 White potatoes are out on the Paleo diet, but celeriac serves as an able replacement, offering the same starchy goodness of potatoes as a counterpoint to the vinegary, spicy dressing. A cousin of celery, celeriac is cultivated for its edible root. You can find large celeriac bulbs in the produce section of the grocery store. Choose small, firm bulbs that are heavy for their size and have no soft spots. Peel them with a vegetable peeler before chopping into cubes.

6 cups peeled and cubed celeriac

2 red onions, chopped

3 celery stalks, chopped

¼ cup apple cider vinegar

1 teaspoon ground celery seed

1 teaspoon sea salt

¼ teaspoon freshly ground black pepper

1 cup Vegetable Stock (page 22)

2 tablespoons arrowroot powder

¼ cup honey

¼ cup chopped fresh parsley

1. In the slow cooker, combine the celeriac, red onions, celery, apple cider vinegar, celery seed, salt, and pepper.

2. In a small bowl, whisk together the Vegetable Stock, arrowroot powder, and honey. Pour the stock mixture over the vegetables, stirring to combine.

3. Cover and cook on low for 8 hours.

4. Stir in the parsley just before serving.

NUTRITION HIGHLIGHT: Celeriac may not be very pretty to look at but it's good for you. It's not as starchy as potatoes, but its mild flavor makes it a great stand-in for stews, soups, and this dish. Celeriac is also a good source of fiber and contains calcium, potassium, and vitamin C.

PER SERVING CALORIES: 146; PROTEIN: 4G; CARBOHYDRATES: 33G; SUGAR: 16G; FAT: 1G; FIBER: 4G; SODIUM: 606MG

Orange-Ginger Beets

PREP TIME: 20 MINUTES / COOK TIME: 8 HOURS

SERVES 6 Beets have a sweet, earthy flavor that blends well with fragrant oranges and the light heat of ginger. While you can use dried ground ginger here, fresh grated ginger root bumps up the flavor. The acid in the orange juice helps preserve the bright red color of the beets and also adds a fresh flavor.

2 pounds beets, peeled and cut into wedges

Juice of 2 oranges

Zest of 1 orange

1 teaspoon grated fresh ginger

1 tablespoon honey

1 tablespoon apple cider vinegar

⅛ teaspoon freshly ground black pepper

Pinch sea salt

1. In the slow cooker, combine the beets, orange juice and zest, ginger, honey, vinegar, pepper, and salt.

2. Cover and cook on low for 8 hours, and serve.

NUTRITION HIGHLIGHT: The bright red color in beets comes from phytonutrients called "betalins," which are antioxidants. Beets are also high in folic acid, manganese, copper, and potassium.

PER SERVING CALORIES: 108; PROTEIN: 3G; CARBOHYDRATES: 25G; SUGAR: 21G; FAT: <1G; FIBER: 5G; SODIUM: 144MG

Sweet AND Spicy Brussels Sprouts

PREP TIME: 10 MINUTES / COOK TIME: 8 HOURS

SERVES 6 When you add sweetness and spiciness to Brussels sprouts, it balances out the bitterness, making them extremely delicious. To prepare the sprouts, simply halve them pole to pole. Feel free to adjust the heat in these sprouts by adding red pepper flakes, if you like them a bit spicier.

Juice and zest of 1 orange

2 tablespoons Orange-Chili-Garlic Sauce (page 28)

¼ cup pure maple syrup

¼ cup apple cider vinegar

1 teaspoon garlic powder

1 teaspoon sea salt

1 pound Brussels sprouts, halved pole to pole

1. In a small bowl, whisk together the orange juice and zest, Orange-Chili-Garlic Sauce, maple syrup, vinegar, garlic powder, and salt.

2. Toss the sauce mixture in the slow cooker with the Brussels sprouts until the sprouts are completely coated.

3. Cover and cook on low for 8 hours, and serve.

NUTRITION HIGHLIGHT: One serving of Brussels sprouts contains more than 100 percent of your recommend daily intake of vitamins C and K. They are also high in folate, a B-complex vitamin that supports good health and is especially important for pregnant women.

PER SERVING CALORIES: 99; PROTEIN: 3G; CARBOHYDRATES: 24G; SUGAR: 16G; FAT: <1G; FIBER: 4G; SODIUM: 367MG

Artichoke AND Swiss Chard Ragout

PREP TIME: 20 MINUTES / COOK TIME: 8 HOURS

SERVES 6 A ragout is a seasoned stew. While it's traditionally made with meat, you can also use veggies to make a hearty and delicious ragout. This works well as a main dish or as a side dish for your meal. It also freezes and reheats well for meals on the go. If you can't find Swiss chard, try substituting it with kale or spinach.

2 (14-ounce) cans artichoke hearts, drained and quartered

1 red onion, chopped

1½ pounds Swiss chard, thick stems removed

1½ teaspoons garlic powder

2 large carrots, peeled and chopped

2 (8-ounce) jars roasted red peppers, drained and chopped

3 cups Vegetable Stock (page 22)

2 tablespoons arrowroot powder

1 teaspoon dried thyme

1 teaspoon sea salt

¼ teaspoon freshly ground black pepper

¼ cup chopped fresh parsley

1. In the slow cooker, combine the artichoke hearts, onion, chard, garlic powder, carrots, and roasted peppers.

2. In a small bowl, whisk together the Vegetable Stock, arrowroot powder, thyme, salt, and pepper. Pour the stock mixture over the vegetables in the slow cooker.

3. Cover and cook on low for 8 hours.

4. Stir in the parsley just before serving.

NUTRITION HIGHLIGHT: Swiss chard is another superfood that's packed with nutrition. It's a rich source of phytonutrients as well as vitamins K, A, and C, iron, calcium, zinc, dietary fiber, and magnesium.

PER SERVING CALORIES: 156; PROTEIN: 10G; CARBOHYDRATES: 31G; SUGAR: 8G; FAT: 1G; FIBER: 11G; SODIUM: 1,259MG

Sweet Potato Curry

PREP TIME: 15 MINUTES / COOK TIME: 9 HOURS

SERVES 6 Sweet potatoes, coconut milk, and warm, fragrant curry make this a delicious main course. Add your favorite seasonal vegetables to make the dish even heartier and more delicious. The nice thing about curry is that it's easy to dump in extra ingredients to make the batch larger or smaller, depending on how many are dining and how much leftovers you want.

4 sweet potatoes, peeled and cubed

1 onion, chopped

2 medium zucchini, chopped

8 ounces shiitake mushrooms, halved

3 cups Vegetable Stock (page 22)

2 cups coconut milk

1 teaspoon garlic powder

1 teaspoon curry powder

1 teaspoon sea salt

½ teaspoon ground ginger

1. In the slow cooker, combine the sweet potatoes, onion, zucchini, mushrooms, Vegetable Stock, coconut milk, garlic powder, curry powder, salt, and ginger.

2. Cover and simmer for 8 hours, and serve.

PORTION ADJUSTMENT: This dish is easy to size up or down for your slow cooker and group size. Plan about ¾ cup of stock and ½ cup of coconut milk per sweet potato, and add as many veggies as you want. For each sweet potato you add to the basic recipe, also add ¼ teaspoon each of garlic powder, curry powder, and salt.

PER SERVING CALORIES: 422; PROTEIN: 8G; CARBOHYDRATES: 57G; SUGAR: 7G; FAT: 20G; FIBER: 10G; SODIUM: 817MG

Spaghetti Squash Marinara

PREP TIME: 10 MINUTES / COOK TIME: 8 HOURS

SERVES 4 If you miss saucy spaghetti, this is the dish for you. Make your Marinara Sauce ahead of time and either refrigerate or freeze it. Then heat it up when your spaghetti squash comes out of the slow cooker.

1 spaghetti squash

1 cup water

4 cups Marinara Sauce (page 31)

1. Poke the spaghetti squash with a fork multiple times.

2. Put the whole squash in the slow cooker with the water.

3. Cover and cook on low for 8 hours.

4. Halve the spaghetti squash pole to pole with a sharp knife. Using a fork, run the tines across the squash to make strands of spaghetti.

5. In a medium saucepan over medium-low heat, heat the Marinara Sauce. Serve over the spaghetti squash "noodles."

A LITTLE LESS PALEO: What's spaghetti and red sauce without a little cheese? Top each plate with 2 tablespoons of grated Parmesan, Romano, or Asiago cheese.

PER SERVING CALORIES: 264; PROTEIN: 5G; CARBOHYDRATES: 45G; SUGAR: 22G; FAT: 8G; FIBER: 7G; SODIUM: 178MG

Honey-Glazed Acorn Squash

PREP TIME: 10 MINUTES / COOK TIME: 8 HOURS

SERVES 6 Sweet honey and spices make this tender acorn squash something special. If you want to save time, you can purchase pre-cubed acorn squash in the produce section of your grocery store, which will limit your active work time to less than 5 minutes—perfect for busy days. You can find Chinese five spice powder in the spice aisle.

Juice of 2 oranges

Zest of 1 orange

¼ cup honey

6 cups acorn squash, peeled, seeded, and cubed

1 tablespoon Chinese five spice powder

1 teaspoon sea salt

1. In a small bowl, whisk the orange juice and zest together with the honey.

2. In the slow cooker, toss the squash with the orange and honey mixture the five spice powder, and the salt.

3. Cover and cook on low for 8 hours, and serve.

PORTION ADJUSTMENT: This recipe is easy to scale for different sizes of slow cookers. Add the juice of 1 orange for every 3 cups of cubed squash, and add about 1 teaspoon of Chinese five spice per 2 cups of squash. Each 3 cups of squash also requires ½ teaspoon of sea salt. Don't add more than the zest of 1 orange, and for smaller batches, just add the zest of half an orange.

PER SERVING CALORIES: 136; PROTEIN: 2G; CARBOHYDRATES: 34G; SUGAR: 17G; FAT: <1G; FIBER: 5G; SODIUM: 317MG

Butternut Squash with Garam Masala

PREP TIME: 10 MINUTES / COOK TIME: 8 HOURS

SERVES 6 With just six ingredients, this squash dish comes together very quickly. You can use any winter squash, or even sweet potatoes, for this recipe if you can't find butternut squash. If you'd like to turn it into a soup, it's easy to purée the squash with 1 cup of coconut milk and 2 or 3 cups of broth to get the desired soup consistency.

6 cups butternut squash

¼ cup pure maple syrup

Juice of 2 oranges

2 tablespoons melted coconut oil

1 tablespoon garam masala

1 teaspoon sea salt

1. In the slow cooker, combine the butternut squash, syrup, orange juice, coconut oil, garam masala, and salt.

2. Cover and cook on low for 8 hours, and serve.

NUTRITION HIGHLIGHT: Adding orange juice brings more than flavor to this recipe. Oranges are high in vitamin C and also contain vitamin A and calcium, while the squash is also an excellent source of vitamin A.

PER SERVING CALORIES: 166; PROTEIN: 2G; CARBOHYDRATES: 32G; SUGAR: 17G; FAT: 5G; FIBER: 4G; SODIUM: 321MG

Eggplant AND Squash Ratatouille

PREP TIME: 20 MINUTES / COOK TIME: 8 HOURS

SERVES 6 The term "ratatouille" is derived from the French term *touiller*. The word means "tossing food," and ratatouille is a tossed-together vegetable dish that is fragrant and flavorful. You can serve it as a side dish, but it is hearty enough to stand on its own. It has a lovely herbal quality that complements the veggies.

1 eggplant, peeled and cubed

1 butternut squash, peeled, seeded, and cubed

2 red bell peppers, seeds and ribs removed, chopped

2 green bell peppers, seeds and ribs removed, chopped

2 zucchini, chopped

1 onion, chopped

1 (14-ounce) can chopped tomatoes, drained

¼ cup extra-virgin olive oil

1 teaspoon dried marjoram

1 teaspoon garlic powder

1 teaspoon sea salt

½ teaspoon dried thyme

¼ teaspoon freshly ground black pepper

¼ cup chopped fresh parsley

1. In the slow cooker, combine the eggplant, butternut squash, bell peppers, zucchini, onion, tomatoes, olive oil, marjoram, garlic powder, salt, thyme, and pepper, stirring to mix well.

2. Cover and cook on low for 8 hours.

3. Stir in the parsley before serving.

PRECOOKING: Eggplant can be a bit bitter, but there's a way to remove the bitter juices. Slice the eggplant and put it in a colander. Sprinkle it with salt and put the colander in the sink. Allow it to sit for 30 minutes. Then wipe away the salt with a paper towel and cube the eggplant for the recipe.

PER SERVING CALORIES: 170; PROTEIN: 4G; CARBOHYDRATES: 22G; SUGAR: 10G; FAT: 9G; FIBER: 7G; SODIUM: 331MG

Winter Vegetable Stew

PREP TIME: 15 MINUTES / COOK TIME: 8 HOURS

SERVES 6 Winter vegetables have a nice hearty quality to them that fills you up when it's cold outside. This stew is made from vegetables commonly available in the winter—winter squash and root vegetables—along with fragrant herbs. The result is a tasty stew that will warm your heart.

4 cups Vegetable Stock (page 22)

2 tablespoons arrowroot powder

1 pound baby carrots

1 pound parsnips, peeled and chopped

1 sweet potato, peeled and cubed

1 acorn squash, peel and seeds removed, cubed

8 shallots, quartered

4 garlic cloves, minced

2 tablespoons coconut oil, melted

1 teaspoon dried thyme

1 teaspoon dried rosemary

1 teaspoon sea salt

¼ teaspoon freshly ground black pepper

¼ cup chopped fresh parsley

1. In a small bowl, whisk together the Vegetable Stock and arrowroot powder.

2. In the slow cooker, combine the carrots, parsnips, sweet potato, squash, shallots, garlic, coconut oil, thyme, rosemary, salt, and pepper. Pour in the broth mixture.

3. Cover and cook on low for 8 hours.

4. Stir in the parsley just before serving.

A LITTLE LESS PALEO: Nothing warms up winter like a bit of wine. Replace 1 cup of the Vegetable Stock with a dry white wine for additional flavor.

PER SERVING CALORIES: 199; PROTEIN: 6G; CARBOHYDRATES: 33G; SUGAR: 9G; FAT: 6G; FIBER: 8G; SODIUM: 898MG

Asian Mushroom Lettuce Wraps

PREP TIME: 20 MINUTES / COOK TIME: 8 HOURS

SERVES 6 Finely chopped mushrooms with Asian spices make a savory filling for lettuce cups. If you have a food processor, you can save time by finely chopping the mushrooms and veggies along with the herbs and spices by pulsing for 10 to 20 one-second pulses. Otherwise, chop your vegetables finely with a knife.

8 ounces cremini mushrooms, finely chopped

8 ounces shiitake mushrooms, finely chopped

1 onion, finely chopped

6 scallions, cut on an angle

6 garlic cloves, minced

1 tablespoon grated fresh ginger

2 tablespoons Orange-Chili-Garlic Sauce (page 28), divided

4 tablespoons chopped fresh cilantro, divided

1 teaspoon Asian fish sauce

1 teaspoon expeller-pressed sesame oil

¼ cup plus 2 tablespoons coconut aminos, divided

½ teaspoon sea salt

1 tablespoon honey

6 large leaves butter lettuce or iceberg lettuce

1. In the slow cooker, combine the mushrooms, onion, scallions, garlic, ginger, 1 tablespoon of Orange-Chili-Garlic Sauce, 2 tablespoons of cilantro, the fish sauce and sesame oil, 2 tablespoons of coconut aminos, and the salt.

2. Cover and simmer on low for 8 hours.

3. In a small bowl, whisk together the remaining 1 tablespoon of Orange-Chili-Garlic Sauce, 2 tablespoons of cilantro, ¼ cup of coconut aminos, and the honey.

4. To serve, spoon the mushroom mixture into the lettuce leaves. Use the honey and coconut aminos mixture as a dipping sauce.

A LITTLE LESS PALEO: Some people find coconut aminos a bit too sweet. Feel free to replace the coconut aminos with an equal amount of gluten-free tamari soy sauce.

PER SERVING CALORIES: 88; PROTEIN: 2G; CARBOHYDRATES: 18G; SUGAR: 6G; FAT: 1G; FIBER: 2G; SODIUM: 383MG

Cabbage Rolls

PREP TIME: 20 MINUTES / COOK TIME: 8 HOURS

SERVES 6 These cabbage rolls are meatless, but meaty mushrooms and almond meal fill in as part of the vegetable stuffing. Napa cabbage is particularly easy to work with because it is pliable, but you can also use green cabbage leaves for the rolls. Blanching the green cabbage leaves (if you use them) for 1 minute in boiling water can help make them more pliable.

2 cups almond meal

1 pound cremini mushrooms, finely chopped

2 onions, finely chopped

2 teaspoons garlic powder, divided

2 teaspoons dried thyme, divided

2 teaspoons sea salt, divided

1 cup Vegetable Stock (page 22)

2 eggs

2 tablespoons coconut oil, melted

1 tablespoon coconut aminos

12 large Napa cabbage leaves

2 (14-ounce) cans crushed tomatoes, undrained

1. In a large bowl, mix together the almond meal, mushrooms, onions, 1 teaspoon of garlic powder, 1 teaspoon of thyme, 1 teaspoon of sea salt, and ¼ teaspoon of pepper with the Vegetable Stock, eggs, coconut oil, and coconut aminos until combined.

2. Spoon the mixture onto the cabbage leaves and roll the cabbage around the filling, tucking in the ends.

3. Place the cabbage rolls, seam-side down, in the slow cooker.

4. In a small bowl, mix together the tomatoes and their juice with the remaining 1 teaspoon of garlic powder, 1 teaspoon of thyme, 1 teaspoon of salt, and ¼ teaspoon of pepper. Pour the tomato mixture over the cabbage rolls.

5. Cover and cook on low for 8 hours, and serve.

PRECOOKING: Browning the mushrooms and onions ahead of time gives a meatier flavor to the filling. To do this, heat the coconut oil in a large sauté pan over medium-high heat. Add the mushrooms and onions. Cook, stirring occasionally, until the mushrooms are browned and have released their liquid, 7 to 10 minutes.

PER SERVING CALORIES: 365; PROTEIN: 17G; CARBOHYDRATES: 30G; SUGAR: 12G; FAT: 22G; FIBER: 14G; SODIUM: 1,045MG

Stuffed Portobello Mushrooms

PREP TIME: 20 MINUTES / COOK TIME: 8 HOURS

SERVES 4 This savory veggie, herb, and almond stuffing makes the perfect filling for meaty, earthy Portobello mushrooms. These mushrooms are large enough that even a single one is a meal. Before using the mushrooms, remove the stems and use the side of a teaspoon to scrape out the black gills underneath. Save the stems for a stock or broth.

2 cups almond meal

1 cup Vegetable Stock (page 22)

2 tablespoons melted coconut oil

1 onion, finely chopped

4 garlic cloves, minced

2 celery stalks, finely chopped

2 carrots, peeled and finely chopped

2 eggs, beaten

1 teaspoon sea salt

¼ teaspoon freshly ground black pepper

4 Portobello mushrooms, stems and gills removed

1. In a medium bowl, mix the almond meal, Vegetable Stock, coconut oil, onion, garlic, celery, carrots, eggs, salt, and pepper.

2. Spoon the mixture into the prepared mushroom caps.

3. Place the mushrooms, stuffed-side up, in the slow cooker.

4. Cover and cook on low for 8 hours, and serve.

PRECOOKING: Sweating the vegetables in the coconut oil adds flavor to the stuffing. To do this, heat the coconut oil in a large sauté pan over medium-high heat. Add the onion, celery, and carrots. Cook, stirring occasionally, until soft, about 5 minutes. Add the garlic and cook, stirring constantly, until it is fragrant—about 30 seconds. Let the vegetables cool, then mix in the almond meal, eggs, salt, pepper, and broth.

PER SERVING CALORIES: 424; PROTEIN: 18G; CARBOHYDRATES: 21G; SUGAR: 5G; FAT: 33G; FIBER: 9G; SODIUM: 720MG

Vegetarian Chili

PREP TIME: 20 MINUTES / COOK TIME: 8 HOURS

SERVES 6 Who needs beans or meat to enjoy chili? This hearty chili is made of veggies, and it's spicy and delicious. Feel free to add any seasonal vegetables into the mix—this is a "dump" meal where it's hard to go wrong with the blend of spices in the chili itself.

2 green bell peppers, seeds and ribs removed, chopped

2 red bell peppers, seeds and ribs removed, chopped

1 (6-ounce) can diced green chiles, drained

2 onions, chopped

3 carrots, peeled and chopped

2 medium zucchini, chopped

8 ounces cremini mushrooms, chopped

2 (14-ounce) cans crushed tomatoes, undrained

2 cups Vegetable Stock (page 22)

1 teaspoon ground cumin

1 teaspoon chili powder

1 teaspoon garlic powder

1 teaspoon dried oregano

1 teaspoon sea salt

½ teaspoon ground coriander

⅛ teaspoon ground cayenne pepper

1. In the slow cooker, combine the bell peppers, chiles, onions, carrots, zucchini, mushrooms, tomatoes and their juice, Vegetable Stock, cumin, chili powder, garlic powder, oregano, salt, coriander, and cayenne.

2. Cover and cook on low for 8 hours, and serve.

A LITTLE LESS PALEO: Replace ¼ cup of the stock with ¼ cup of whiskey for a tasty, boozy chili. Top the chili with grated Cheddar cheese, a dollop of sour cream, and chopped avocados.

PER SERVING CALORIES: 224; PROTEIN: 11G; CARBOHYDRATES: 45G; SUGAR: 26G; FAT: 3G; FIBER: 16G; SODIUM: 885MG

Hearty Mushroom Stew

PREP TIME: 15 MINUTES / COOK TIME: 8 HOURS

SERVES 4 Mushrooms are deliciously meaty, so they make a delicious and hearty stew. Using dried porcini mushrooms in stock lends an even deeper mushroom flavor to the stew. If you can't find dried porcinis, you can use any type of dried mushrooms you can find, and they will flavor the stock just as well.

2 ounces dried porcini mushrooms

4 cups Vegetable Stock (page 22)

2 tablespoons arrowroot powder

1 tablespoon Dijon mustard

8 ounces cremini mushrooms, quartered

4 Portobello mushrooms, stems and gills removed, chopped

8 ounces button mushrooms, quartered

2 carrots, peeled and chopped

1 red onion, chopped

1 teaspoon dried rosemary

1 teaspoon dried thyme

1 teaspoon garlic powder

1 teaspoon sea salt

¼ teaspoon freshly ground black pepper

Pinch red pepper flakes

¼ cup chopped fresh parsley

1. The night before you make your dish, in a large bowl, soak the dried mushrooms in the Vegetable Stock overnight.

2. Remove the mushrooms from the stock, and add them to the slow cooker.

3. Whisk the stock with the arrowroot powder and the Dijon mustard.

4. In the slow cooker, combine the cremini mushrooms, Portobello mushrooms, button mushrooms, carrots, onion, rosemary, thyme, garlic powder, salt, pepper, red pepper flakes, and the stock mixture with the dried mushrooms.

5. Cover and cook on low for 8 hours.

6. Stir in the parsley before serving.

SEASONAL INGREDIENTS: Chanterelle mushrooms are available in the fall. These hearty mushrooms are an excellent addition to this stew, adding a rich, meaty flavor and texture. Replace any or all the mushrooms with chanterelles when they are available.

PER SERVING CALORIES: 188; PROTEIN: 16G; CARBOHYDRATES: 26G; SUGAR: 6G; FAT: 2G; FIBER: 7G; SODIUM: 1,037MG

Vegetable Pot Pie
WITH Almond Crust

PREP TIME: 20 MINUTES / COOK TIME: 8 HOURS

SERVES 6 Almond meal serves as the basis for the crust of this slow cooker pie. Under the rich crust are savory veggies in a stock fragranced with delicious tarragon, which has a delicate flavor and aroma. Feel free to substitute any veggies you like in this pie, with the exception of cruciferous ones such as cabbage, broccoli, and cauliflower, which will impart bitter flavors.

1 pound cremini mushrooms, quartered

1 onion, chopped

3 large carrots, peeled and chopped

2 red bell peppers, seeded and chopped

2 celery stalks, chopped

1 teaspoon dried tarragon

3 cups Vegetable Stock (page 22)

2 tablespoons arrowroot powder

2 teaspoons sea salt, divided

¼ teaspoon freshly ground black pepper

2 cups almond meal

1 teaspoon baking soda

½ cup coconut oil, melted

4 large eggs, beaten

1 tablespoon honey

1. In the slow cooker, combine the mushrooms, onion, carrots, bell peppers, and celery.

2. In a small bowl, whisk together the tarragon, Vegetable Stock, arrowroot powder, 1 teaspoon of salt, and the pepper. Pour the stock mixture over the vegetables.

3. In a large bowl, stir to combine the almond meal, baking soda, remaining 1 teaspoon of salt, coconut oil, eggs, and honey until well mixed.

4. Drop the almond meal mixture by the spoonful on top of the vegetable mixture.

5. Cover and cook on low for 8 hours, and serve.

NUTRITION HIGHLIGHT: Arrowroot powder comes from the roots of tropical plants in South America. Unlike cornstarch, arrowroot thickens without GMOs or grains. It is made by grating the roots, soaking them in water, and then dehydrating the starch. It's an excellent natural alternative to grain-based thickeners.

PER SERVING CALORIES: 355; PROTEIN: 12G; CARBOHYDRATES: 19G; SUGAR: 9G; FAT: 27G; FIBER: 4G; SODIUM: 1,303MG

Cauliflower Curry

PREP TIME: 10 MINUTES / COOK TIME: 8 HOURS

SERVES 6 Cauliflower makes a lovely base for a curry. Its mild flavor takes on the spices in the fragrant curry sauce. Canned tomatoes make the prep super quick, and the spinach adds color and nutrients. This freezes well, so you can make a large batch and store some for future meals, if you like.

2 heads cauliflower, broken into florets

8 ounces shiitake mushrooms, halved

1 onion, chopped

1 pound baby spinach

2 cups Vegetable Stock (page 22)

1 (14-ounce) can crushed tomatoes, undrained

2 cups coconut milk, plus ¼ cup for serving (optional)

2 teaspoons curry powder

1 teaspoon garlic powder

1 teaspoon sea salt

½ teaspoon ground ginger

1. In the slow cooker, combine the cauliflower, mushrooms, onion, spinach, Vegetable Stock, tomatoes and their juice, coconut milk, curry powder, garlic powder, salt, and ginger.

2. Cover and simmer on low for 8 hours.

3. Drizzle with coconut milk as a garnish, if desired, and serve.

NUTRITION HIGHLIGHT: Spinach is another superfood that is a nutritional powerhouse. It's loaded with antioxidants, including vitamin C, and it's a rich source of iron, vitamins A and K, folate, manganese, calcium, and magnesium.

PER SERVING CALORIES: 295; PROTEIN: 10G; CARBOHYDRATES: 25G; SUGAR: 11G; FAT: 20G; FIBER: 9G; SODIUM: 884MG

Mexican Cauliflower "Rice"

PREP TIME: 20 MINUTES / COOK TIME: 8 HOURS

SERVES 6 If you miss rice, you may enjoy this version, made with grated cauliflower flavored with Mexican herbs and spices. You can have it alone or combine it with ground beef, shredded beef, shredded pork, or other meats. Grating the cauliflower gives it a rice-like texture. If you have a food processor, you can also pulse the cauliflower florets in the processor for 10 one-second pulses, or until it resembles rice.

2 heads cauliflower, grated

1 onion, chopped

1 (14-ounce) can tomatoes and peppers

1 teaspoon ground cumin

1 teaspoon chili powder

1 teaspoon garlic powder

1 teaspoon dried oregano

1 teaspoon sea salt

Dash ground cayenne pepper

Zest of 1 lime

Juice of 1 lime

¼ cup chopped fresh cilantro

1. In the slow cooker, combine the cauliflower, onion, tomatoes and peppers, cumin, chili powder, garlic powder, oregano, salt, cayenne, and lime zest.

2. Cover and cook on low for 8 hours.

3. Stir in the lime juice and cilantro just before serving.

A LITTLE LESS PALEO: Top the rice with grated Cotija cheese (a flavorful, hard cow's milk cheese) in the last 30 minutes of cooking, and serve the rice topped with Mexican crema (which is similar to sour cream).

PER SERVING CALORIES: 57; PROTEIN: 3G; CARBOHYDRATES: 12G; SUGAR: 7G; FAT: <1G; FIBER: 4G; SODIUM: 570MG

Cauliflower AND Mushroom Bolognese

PREP TIME: 20 MINUTES / COOK TIME: 8 HOURS

SERVES 6 Traditional Bolognese is an Italian meat-based sauce. In this dish, cauliflower and mushroom offer meaty flavor and texture in a lighter, vegan Paleo version. Serve it on top of any steamed veggies, or make zucchini ribbon noodles by using a carrot peeler to cut the zucchini into long strips.

1 head cauliflower, broken into florets

1 pound cremini mushrooms, finely chopped

1 red onion, chopped

2 (14-ounce) cans crushed tomatoes, drained

¼ cup Vegetable Stock (page 22)

1 teaspoon garlic powder

1 teaspoon dried oregano

1 teaspoon sea salt

Pinch red pepper flakes

¼ cup chopped fresh basil

1. In the slow cooker, combine the cauliflower, mushrooms, onion, tomatoes, Vegetable Stock, garlic powder, oregano, salt, and red pepper flakes.

2. Cover and cook on low for 8 hours.

3. Using a potato masher, lightly mash the sauce to break up the cauliflower.

4. Stir in the basil just before serving.

NUTRITION HIGHLIGHT: Basil has a pleasant, bright herbal taste and fragrance, and it's also very healthy. According to World's Healthiest Foods, basil is anti-inflammatory and antibacterial, and it's rich in vitamin K, so feel free to use this flavorful herb liberally in your cooking.

PER SERVING CALORIES: 96; PROTEIN: 7G; CARBOHYDRATES: 18G; SUGAR: 11G; FAT: <1G; FIBER: 6G; SODIUM: 617MG

Veggie Lasagna

PREP TIME: 20 MINUTES / COOK TIME: 8 HOURS

SERVES 6 While a traditional lasagna has layers of meat, cheese, and noodles, this vegan Paleo version lightens it up and relies on lots of healthy vegetables and flavorful herbs. Greasing the inside of the slow cooker will help keep the lasagna from sticking as it cooks. Make the Bolognese ahead of time to make this recipe even quicker.

Paleo-friendly fat or oil, for greasing

1 recipe Cauliflower and Mushroom
    Bolognese (page 108), divided

2 eggplants, thinly sliced, divided

1 pound frozen spinach, thawed, divided

1. Using your favorite Paleo-friendly fat or oil, grease the slow cooker insert.

2. Spread a quarter of the Bolognese on the bottom of the slow cooker.

3. Add a layer of eggplant, then half the spinach.

4. Add another quarter of the Bolognese, and then a layer of the eggplant followed by the remaining half of the spinach.

5. Add another quarter of the Bolognese, and a final layer of eggplant. Pour the remaining quarter of Bolognese over the eggplant.

6. Cover and cook on low for 8 hours, and serve.

PRECOOKING: To make the lasagna less watery, put the eggplant slices in a colander in the sink and sprinkle them with salt. Allow the water to drain from the eggplant for an hour, and then wipe away the salt with a paper towel. Wring the spinach in a clean kitchen towel to remove excess water.

PER SERVING CALORIES: 159; PROTEIN: 11G; CARBOHYDRATES: 32G; SUGAR: 17G; FAT: 2G; FIBER: 14G; SODIUM: 680MG

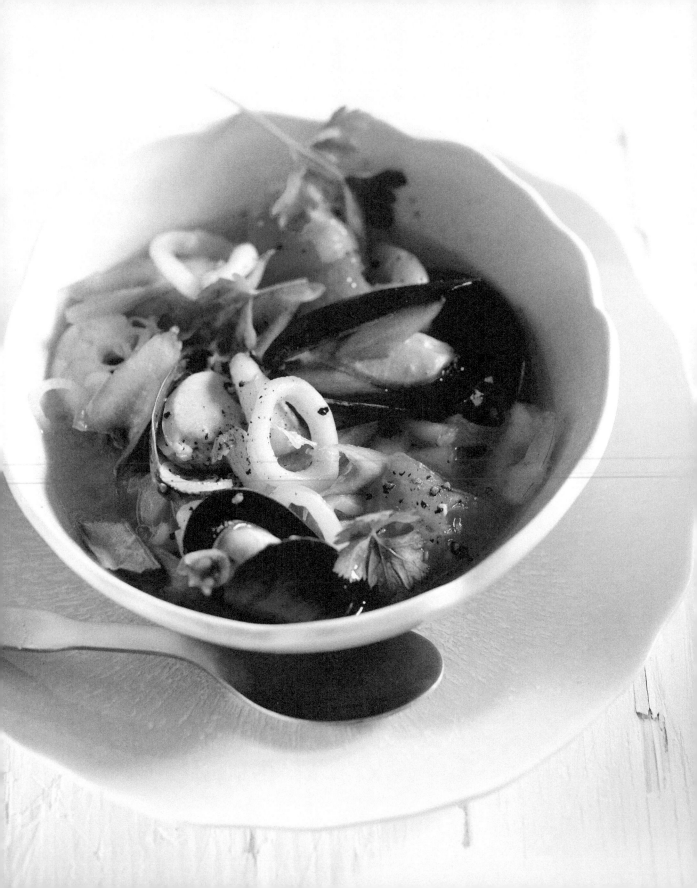

CHAPTER SEVEN

Seafood and Poultry

Crab AND Lemon Cauliflower "Rice"

PREP TIME: 10 MINUTES / COOK TIME: 8½ HOURS

SERVES 4 Lemon and crab is a classic flavor combination. The acidity of the lemon cuts through the rich, fishy sweetness of the crab. You can find fresh, shelled lump crab meat in the seafood section of your grocery store. Drain and pick over the meat to remove any bits of shell before adding to the recipe.

2 heads cauliflower, grated

Juice of 2 lemons

Zest of 1 lemon

1 onion, chopped

3 carrots, peeled and chopped

2 red bell peppers, seeded and chopped

2 cups Fish Stock (page 24)

1 teaspoon sea salt

¼ teaspoon freshly ground black pepper

Pinch red pepper flakes

1 pound lump crab meat

¼ cup chopped fresh parsley

1. In the slow cooker, combine the cauliflower, lemon juice, lemon zest, onion, carrots, bell peppers, Fish Stock, salt, pepper, and pepper flakes.

2. Cover and cook on low for 8 hours.

3. Stir in the crab meat and parsley.

4. Cover and cook for an additional 30 minutes, or until the crab is warmed through, and serve.

A LITTLE LESS PALEO: Green peas are legumes and thus technically not allowed on a Paleo diet, although some Paleo dieters eat them occasionally. If you'd like to add a fresh hint of green to this dish, stir in some fresh green peas along with the crab and parsley for the last 30 minutes of cooking.

PER SERVING CALORIES: 184; PROTEIN: 23G; CARBOHYDRATES: 21G; SUGAR: 9G; FAT: 10G; FIBER: 6G; SODIUM: 1,567MG

Halibut WITH Lemon AND Capers

PREP TIME: 10 MINUTES / COOK TIME: 8 HOURS

SERVES 6 While the recipe calls for halibut, you can add any white fish fillets to this recipe. The briny capers add saltiness, while the lemon is acidic and pairs well with the richness of the halibut. Remove the skin from the halibut and cut it into 1-inch pieces so it cooks quickly.

Juice of 2 lemons

Zest of 1 lemon

¼ cup capers, drained

6 cups Fish Stock (page 24)

3 carrots, peeled and chopped

2 red bell peppers, seeds and ribs removed, chopped

2 zucchini, chopped

½ teaspoon garlic powder

½ teaspoon sea salt

¼ teaspoon freshly ground black pepper

1½ pounds halibut fillets, skin and bones removed, cut into 1-inch cubes

¼ cup chopped fresh parsley

1. In the slow cooker, combine the lemon juice, lemon zest, capers, Fish Stock, carrots, bell peppers, zucchini, garlic powder, salt, and pepper.

2. Cover and cook on low for 7½ hours.

3. Add the halibut. Cover and cook on high for an additional 30 minutes, or until the halibut is cooked.

4. Stir in the parsley just before serving.

> **A LITTLE LESS PALEO:** White wine blends beautifully with halibut, and butter adds richness. Replace 1 cup of the broth with an equal amount of white wine, and add 2 tablespoons of grass-fed butter when you add the parsley, stirring until the butter melts.

PER SERVING CALORIES: 190; PROTEIN: 32G; CARBOHYDRATES: 8G; SUGAR: 4G; FAT: 3G; FIBER: 2G; SODIUM: 1,208MG

Cod WITH Coconut, Lemongrass, AND Shiitake Mushrooms

PREP TIME: 20 MINUTES / COOK TIME: 8 HOURS

SERVES 6 Lemongrass has a light, citrusy flavor that pairs well with cod. The shiitake mushrooms add meatiness, and the coconut adds a creamy touch of richness that gives this dish a classic Thai flavor profile. Remove the skin and bones from the cod before adding it, and chop it into 1-inch pieces to facilitate quick cooking.

4 cups Fish Stock (page 24)

2 cups coconut milk

1 leek (white and green parts), sliced

1 pound shiitake mushrooms, sliced

3 lemongrass stalks, finely chopped

1 tablespoon grated fresh ginger

1 tablespoon Orange-Chili-Garlic Sauce (page 28)

1 teaspoon Asian fish sauce

1 teaspoon garlic powder

1 teaspoon sea salt

¼ teaspoon freshly ground black pepper

1½ pounds cod fillets, bones and skin removed, cut into 1-inch cubes

¼ cup chopped fresh cilantro

1. In the slow cooker, combine the Fish Stock, coconut milk, leeks, mushrooms, lemongrass, ginger, Orange-Chili-Garlic Sauce, fish sauce, garlic powder, salt, and pepper.

2. Cover and cook on low for 7½ hours.

3. Stir in the cod. Cover and cook on high for an additional 30 minutes, or until the cod is cooked.

4. Stir in the cilantro just before serving.

NUTRITION HIGHLIGHT: Cod is a cold, deepwater fish. It is an excellent source of lean protein and provides a hefty dose of vitamin B12 per serving, as well as iodine and selenium.

PER SERVING CALORIES: 386; PROTEIN: 33G; CARBOHYDRATES: 19; SUGAR: 7G; FAT: 21G; FIBER: 7G; SODIUM: 1,201MG

Ginger-Poached Cod

PREP TIME: 10 MINUTES / COOK TIME: 8 HOURS

SERVES 6 Poaching cod and vegetables in this ginger broth gives the mild cod a delicious ginger/peppery bite. Don't toss the broth—serve it spooned around the cod and vegetables to bump up the flavor of this light dish. This is a delicious, healthy recipe to serve when you don't want heavy food weighing you down.

8 cups Ginger-Poultry Broth (page 25)

3 large zucchini (or summer squash), chopped

2 red bell peppers, seeds and ribs removed, chopped

3 large carrots, peeled and chopped

1 onion, chopped

1 tablespoon grated fresh ginger

1 teaspoon garlic powder

Zest of 1 lime

1 teaspoon sea salt

¼ teaspoon freshly ground black pepper

1½ pounds cod fillets, skin and bones removed, cut into 1-inch pieces

Juice of 2 limes

1. In the slow cooker, combine the Ginger-Poultry Broth, zucchini, red peppers, carrots, onion, ginger, garlic powder, lime zest, salt, and pepper.

2. Cover and cook on low for 7½ hours.

3. Stir in the cod and lime juice.

4. Cover and cook on high for an additional 30 minutes, or until the cod is cooked, and serve.

> **PRECOOKING:** For a deeper flavor, cook the onion in 2 tablespoons of coconut oil for 5 minutes, stirring occasionally, and then add to the slow cooker.

PER SERVING CALORIES: 236; PROTEIN: 35G; CARBOHYDRATES: 17; SUGAR: 8G; FAT: 3G; FIBER: 4G; SODIUM: 1,462MG

Seafood Stew

PREP TIME: 15 MINUTES / COOK TIME: 8 HOURS

SERVES 6 This is a rich, brothy stew that has a tasty lemon and herbal flavor. Feel free to pick your own favorite seafoods for this stew. Just make sure you cut the seafood into small enough pieces that will cook quickly in the hot broth when you add them. You can also switch up the vegetables, choosing those that are in season.

6 cups Fish Stock (page 24), divided

1 pound pearl onions, peeled

8 ounces cremini mushrooms, halved

3 roma tomatoes, chopped

1 celeriac bulb, peeled and cubed

1 fennel bulb, chopped

2 celery stalks, chopped

3 large carrots, peeled and chopped

1 teaspoon dried tarragon

1 teaspoon sea salt

¼ teaspoon freshly ground black pepper

Juice of 1 lemon

2 tablespoons arrowroot powder

6 ounces cod fillet, skin and bones removed, cut into 1-inch pieces

6 ounces salmon fillet, skin and bones removed, cut into 1-inch pieces

8 ounces cooked baby shrimp

8 ounces mussels, cleaned and debearded

¼ cup chopped fresh parsley

Zest of 1 lemon

1. In the slow cooker, combine 5 cups of Fish Stock with the pearl onions, mushrooms, tomatoes, celeriac, fennel, celery, carrots, tarragon, salt, and pepper.

2. Cover and cook on low for 7½ hours.

3. In a small bowl, whisk together the lemon juice, remaining 1 cup of stock, and arrowroot powder.

4. Add them to the slow cooker, along with the cod, salmon, shrimp, and mussels.

5. Turn the slow cooker up to high and cook for an additional 30 minutes, or until the fish is cooked.

6. Stir in the parsley and lemon zest just before serving.

NUTRITION HIGHLIGHT: Salmon is one of the fattier seafoods. It is a rich source of omega-3 fatty acids as well as plenty of vitamin B12, vitamin D, and selenium.

PER SERVING CALORIES: 287; PROTEIN: 34G; CARBOHYDRATES: 30; SUGAR: 9G; FAT: 7G; FIBER: 6G; SODIUM: 1,745MG

Jambalaya

PREP TIME: 20 MINUTES / COOK TIME: 8 HOURS

SERVES 8 This rich, thick stew is packing heat. Loaded with the flavor of onions, garlic, peppers, and andouille sausage, along with the sweetness of shrimp, it's like a party in your mouth. This is a dish that freezes very well and lends itself to doubling up on a batch, so you can stock your freezer with Paleo meals to go.

1 pound andouille sausage, sliced

1 pound medium shrimp, peeled and deveined

2 (14-ounce) cans crushed tomatoes, undrained

2 cups Fish Stock (page 24)

2 green bell peppers, seeds and ribs removed, chopped

2 red bell peppers, seeds and ribs removed, chopped

2 large carrots, chopped

1 onion, chopped

2 jalapeño peppers, seeded and chopped

1 teaspoon ground smoked paprika

1 teaspoon garlic powder

1 teaspoon Cajun seasoning mix

1 teaspoon sea salt

¼ teaspoon freshly ground black pepper

⅛ teaspoon ground cayenne pepper

1. In the slow cooker, combine the sausage, shrimp, tomatoes and their juice, Fish Stock, bell peppers, carrots, onion, jalapeños, paprika, garlic powder, Cajun seasoning, salt, black pepper, and cayenne.

2. Cover and cook on low for 8 hours, and serve.

NUTRITION HIGHLIGHT: This jambalaya is packed with antioxidants, including carotenoids from the bell peppers and carrots and lycopene from the tomatoes. It's a great way to fight oxidative stress while enjoying delicious, spicy food.

PER SERVING CALORIES: 325; PROTEIN: 28G; CARBOHYDRATES: 17; SUGAR: 9G; FAT: 17G; FIBER: 5G; SODIUM: 1,449MG

Shrimp Creole

PREP TIME: 20 MINUTES / COOK TIME: 8 HOURS

SERVES 6 This Louisiana French Creole specialty uses the "holy trinity" of Cajun cooking: onions, celery, and bell peppers. Plenty of cayenne pepper adds heat, but feel free to adjust the heat to your liking. This is fragrant as it cooks, so your kitchen will smell delicious. To save time, buy shrimp that has already been peeled and deveined.

2 onions, diced

2 celery stalks, diced

2 green bell peppers, seeds and ribs removed, diced

2 (14-ounce) cans crushed tomatoes, undrained

1 tablespoon coconut aminos

1 tablespoon honey

1 teaspoon chili powder

1 teaspoon sea salt

¼ teaspoon ground cayenne pepper

⅛ teaspoon freshly ground black pepper

1½ pounds medium shrimp, peeled and deveined

6 scallions, chopped

1. In the slow cooker, combine the onions, celery, bell peppers, tomatoes and their juice, coconut aminos, honey, chili powder, salt, cayenne, and black pepper.

2. Cover and cook on low for 7½ hours.

3. Stir in the shrimp. Cover and cook on high for an additional 30 minutes.

4. Stir in the scallions just before serving.

PRECOOKING: To add a depth of flavor, brown the onions, celery, and peppers in 2 tablespoons of coconut oil. Cook them over medium-high heat for 5 to 7 minutes, stirring occasionally until browned, and then add them to the slow cooker.

PER SERVING CALORIES: 258; PROTEIN: 34G; CARBOHYDRATES: 25; SUGAR: 15G; FAT: 3G; FIBER: 7G; SODIUM: 1,603MG

Shrimp Fajitas

PREP TIME: 15 MINUTES / COOK TIME: 8 HOURS

SERVES 6 Fajitas are a Tex-Mex food, originally made using skirt steak. However, as the dish has grown in popularity, chefs have used seafood, pork, poultry, and even vegetables to make fajitas. Shrimp, peppers, and onion are the basis for these fajitas. Using lettuce as tortillas eliminates grain-based wraps. Serve with Cooked Salsa (page 29) for additional flavor.

3 cups Vegetable Stock (page 22)

3 green bell peppers, seeds and ribs removed, sliced

3 onions, sliced

Zest of 1 lime

Juice of 2 limes

1 teaspoon ground cumin

1 teaspoon chili powder

1 teaspoon garlic powder

1 teaspoon ground coriander

1 teaspoon sea salt

1½ pounds shrimp, peeled and deveined

¼ cup chopped fresh cilantro

12 lettuce leaves

1 cup Cooked Salsa (page 29)

1 avocado, peeled, pitted, and cubed

1. In the slow cooker, combine the Vegetable Stock, peppers, onions, lime zest, lime juice, cumin, chili powder, garlic powder, coriander, and salt.

2. Cover and cook on low for 7½ hours.

3. Stir in the shrimp. Cover and cook on high for an additional 30 minutes, or until the shrimp is cooked through.

4. Stir in the cilantro.

5. Serve wrapped in the lettuce leaves, topped with the Cooked Salsa and the avocado.

A LITTLE LESS PALEO: Serve the fajitas with sour cream and some shredded Monterey Jack cheese.

PER SERVING CALORIES: 250; PROTEIN: 30G; CARBOHYDRATES: 16; SUGAR: 6G; FAT: 9G; FIBER: 6G; SODIUM: 1,222MG

Scampi

PREP TIME: 20 MINUTES / COOK TIME: 8 HOURS

SERVES 6 Traditionally served over pasta, shrimp scampi is a tasty combination of lemon, garlic, olive oil, shrimp, and herbs. This version calls for the quick addition of zucchini noodles at the end. To make the noodles, use a vegetable peeler or spiralizer to cut thin ribbons of the zucchini. If you'd like, use a sharp knife to cut the zucchini ribbons into thinner strips.

8 garlic cloves, minced

¼ cup extra-virgin olive oil

Juice of 2 lemons

Zest of 1 lemon

2 onions, sliced

1 red bell pepper, ribs and seeds removed, chopped

4 cups Fish Stock (page 24)

½ teaspoon sea salt

⅛ teaspoon freshly ground black pepper

Pinch red pepper flakes

1½ pounds shrimp, peeled and deveined

3 large zucchini, cut into noodles

¼ cup chopped fresh basil

1. In the slow cooker, combine the garlic, olive oil, lemon juice and zest, onions, bell pepper, Fish Stock, salt, pepper, and red pepper flakes.

2. Cover and cook on low for 7½ hours.

3. Stir in the shrimp and zucchini noodles. Cover and cook on high for an additional 30 minutes, or until the shrimp is cooked through.

4. Stir in the basil just before serving.

A LITTLE LESS PALEO: Traditional scampi also uses white wine. Replace 1 cup of the Fish Stock with 1 cup of white wine. Sprinkle on a little grated Parmesan cheese before serving.

PER SERVING CALORIES: 265; PROTEIN: 29G; CARBOHYDRATES: 15G; SUGAR: 6G; FAT: 11G; FIBER: 5G; SODIUM: 452MG

Whole Roasted Chicken

PREP TIME: 15 MINUTES / COOK TIME: 8 HOURS

SERVES 4 If you're looking for an easy way to roast a chicken, this is it. Stuffing the cavity with herbs flavors the meat, and the chicken's juices drip downward to the vegetables to flavor those as well. It's an easy way to have Sunday dinner any night of the week, no matter how busy your schedule is.

1 celeriac bulb, peeled and cubed

1 fennel bulb, sliced

8 ounces baby carrots

8 shallots, peeled and quartered

1 teaspoon smoked paprika

1 teaspoon garlic powder

1 teaspoon onion powder

1 teaspoon dried thyme

1 teaspoon sea salt

⅛ teaspoon freshly ground black pepper

1 whole chicken

1 lemon, cut in half

1 onion, cut in half

2 fresh thyme sprigs

2 fresh rosemary sprigs

1. In the slow cooker, combine the celeriac, fennel, carrots, and shallots.

2. In a small bowl, mix the paprika, garlic powder, onion powder, thyme, salt, and pepper. Rub the spice mixture all over the outside of the chicken.

3. Stuff the chicken cavity with the lemon halves, onion halves, thyme, and rosemary sprigs. Place the chicken, breast-side up, on top of the vegetables in the slow cooker.

4. Cover and cook on low for 8 hours, and serve.

SEASONAL INGREDIENTS: You can change the vegetables according to the season. For example, in the spring and summer, add an array of summer squash, such as zucchini and pattypan squash. In the winter, try winter squash. In spring, you can add asparagus.

PER SERVING CALORIES: 254; PROTEIN: 35G; CARBOHYDRATES: 19G; SUGAR: 6G; FAT: 4G; FIBER: 5G; SODIUM: 656MG

Jerk Chicken

PREP TIME: 10 MINUTES / COOK TIME: 8 HOURS

QP

SERVES 4 Jerk cooking comes from Jamaica, and it refers to a certain way of cooking and seasoning meat. Typically the meat is marinated in a spicy marinade with Scotch bonnet peppers, which are an extremely hot pepper, and then slow smoked. This recipe substitutes a dry rub for the marinade and slow cooking for smoking, but the flavors are similar.

2 sweet potatoes, cubed

1 teaspoon garlic powder

1 teaspoon onion powder

1 teaspoon coconut sugar

1 teaspoon sea salt

½ teaspoon ground smoked paprika

½ teaspoon ground allspice

¼ teaspoon ground cayenne pepper

¼ teaspoon freshly ground black pepper

¼ teaspoon ground nutmeg

Pinch ground cinnamon

1 whole chicken, cut into parts (or 1 pound of cut chicken parts)

1. In the bottom of the slow cooker, arrange the sweet potatoes.

2. In a small bowl, mix the garlic powder, onion powder, coconut sugar, salt, paprika, allspice, cayenne, black pepper, nutmeg, and cinnamon.

3. Rub the spice mixture onto the chicken pieces. Arrange the pieces in the slow cooker on top of the sweet potatoes.

4. Cover and cook on low for 8 hours, and serve.

PRECOOKING: Brown the spice-rubbed chicken pieces in a large pan over medium heat in 2 tablespoons of your favorite Paleo fat, about 3 minutes per side, before adding them to the slow cooker. This renders some of the fat in the chicken skin and adds flavor.

PER SERVING CALORIES: 315; PROTEIN: 35G; CARBOHYDRATES: 34G; SUGAR: 2G; FAT: 4G; FIBER: 5G; SODIUM: 550MG

Bacon-Wrapped Drumsticks

PREP TIME: 10 MINUTES / COOK TIME: 8 HOURS

SERVES 6 Nothing makes chicken taste better than smoky bacon. This recipe is super easy, and it's always popular at potlucks. Use thin-cut bacon so it cooks through. Serve with steamed veggies, cauliflower mash, or just salad for a healthy, complete meal. This also makes an excellent meal on the go, as it reheats quickly.

12 chicken drumsticks

12 slices thin-cut bacon

1. Wrap each drumstick in bacon, and put it in the slow cooker.

2. Cover and cook on low for 8 hours, and serve.

PORTION ADJUSTMENT: This recipe is super easy to size up or down. Just use as many drumsticks as you want and as much room as you have in the slow cooker. Alternatively, you can put the drumsticks in a baking pan and roast at 350°F for 1 hour.

PER SERVING CALORIES: 202; PROTEIN: 30G; CARBOHYDRATES: 0G; SUGAR: 0G; FAT: 8G; FIBER: 0G; SODIUM: 254MG

Barbecue Chicken Drumsticks

PREP TIME: 10 MINUTES / COOK TIME: 8 HOURS

SERVES 6 A simple, sticky barbecue sauce adds smoke, sweetness, and flavor to chicken drumsticks (or any other chicken parts you choose). Serve it alongside German-Style Celeriac (page 87) for a tasty picnic-style dinner. You can even make extra barbecue sauce and save it for later use.

1 (6-ounce) can tomato paste

¼ cup pure maple syrup

¼ cup apple cider vinegar

1 teaspoon smoked paprika

1 teaspoon garlic powder

1 teaspoon chili powder

1 teaspoon onion powder

1 teaspoon sea salt

½ teaspoon liquid smoke

½ teaspoon ground cumin

12 chicken drumsticks

1. In a small bowl, whisk together the tomato paste, maple syrup, cider vinegar, smoked paprika, garlic powder, chili powder, onion powder, salt, liquid smoke, and cumin.

2. Arrange the drumsticks in the slow cooker, and pour the sauce over the top.

3. Cover and cook on low for 8 hours, and serve.

A LITTLE LESS PALEO: Replace the apple cider vinegar with an equal amount of whiskey for a deeper, slightly boozy flavor.

PER SERVING CALORIES: 221; PROTEIN: 27G; CARBOHYDRATES: 15G; SUGAR: 12G; FAT: 6G; FIBER: 2G; SODIUM: 353MG

Maple-Glazed Chicken Thighs

PREP TIME: 10 MINUTES / COOK TIME: 8 HOURS

SERVES 6 This is another very quick prep chicken recipe. You can either use skin-on, bone-in thighs or bone-less skinless thighs—it's up to you. The maple glaze is sweet and a little spicy, which complements the rich flavor of the chicken perfectly. When served with a veggie side, it makes a tasty meal.

12 chicken thighs

¼ cup pure maple syrup

¼ cup coconut aminos

2 tablespoons tomato paste

1 teaspoon garlic powder

½ teaspoon sea salt

⅛ teaspoon freshly ground black pepper

Dash ground cayenne pepper

1. In the bottom of the slow cooker, arrange the chicken thighs.

2. In a small bowl, whisk together the maple syrup, coconut aminos, tomato paste, garlic powder, salt, pepper, and cayenne. Pour the mixture over the thighs.

3. Cover and cook on low for 8 hours, and serve.

A LITTLE LESS PALEO: You can replace the tomato paste with sugar-free ketchup here, and if you like, you can use gluten-free tamari soy sauce in place of the coconut aminos.

PER SERVING CALORIES: 310; PROTEIN: 30G; CARBOHYDRATES: 12G; SUGAR: 9G; FAT: 14G; FIBER: 0G; SODIUM: 350MG

Lemon-Thyme Chicken

PREP TIME: 15 MINUTES / COOK TIME: 8 HOURS

SERVES 6 The combination of lemon and thyme is classic. The lemon adds brightness and acidity, while thyme has a woody, herbal taste to rich chicken thighs. Although this recipe calls for thighs, you can use any chicken pieces you prefer. The chicken's juices drip down to season the vegetables underneath.

8 ounces cremini mushrooms, quartered

2 large zucchini, chopped

8 ounces pearl onions, peeled

Juice of 2 lemons

Zest of 1 lemon

2 cups Bone Broth (page 26) made with chicken bones

2 tablespoons arrowroot powder

1 teaspoon dried thyme

1 teaspoon garlic powder

1 teaspoon sea salt

⅛ teaspoon freshly ground black pepper

12 chicken thighs

1. In the slow cooker, combine the mushrooms, zucchini, and onions.

2. In a small bowl, whisk together the lemon juice and zest with the Bone Broth, arrowroot, thyme, garlic powder, salt, and pepper.

3. Arrange the chicken thighs on top of the vegetables, and pour the lemon juice mixture over the top.

4. Cover and cook on low for 8 hours, and serve.

A LITTLE LESS PALEO: White wine adds delicious flavor to this dish. Replace 1 cup of broth with an equal amount of white wine.

PER SERVING CALORIES: 230; PROTEIN: 30G; CARBOHYDRATES: 14G; SUGAR: 5G; FAT: 6G; FIBER: 3G; SODIUM: 655MG

Chicken AND Mushroom Stew

PREP TIME: 15 MINUTES / COOK TIME: 8 HOURS

SERVES 6 Earthy mushrooms complement the chicken and herbs in this simple yet flavorful stew. Tarragon adds delicate flavor and fragrance, while orange is a surprising and complex addition. Feel free to use any type of chicken meat you like, although thigh meat tends to be a bit fattier, so it works better in the slow cooker than white meat.

2 ounces bacon, chopped

2 red onions, chopped

1 pound cremini mushrooms, quartered

8 ounces baby carrots

3 zucchini, chopped

1 teaspoon dried tarragon

Juice of 2 oranges

Zest of 1 orange

2 cups Bone Broth (page 26) made with chicken bones

2 tablespoons arrowroot powder

1 teaspoon sea salt

¼ teaspoon freshly ground black pepper

1½ pounds chicken thigh meat, cut into 1-inch pieces

¼ cup chopped fresh parsley

1. In the slow cooker, combine the bacon, onions, mushrooms, carrots, zucchini, tarragon, orange juice, and orange zest.

2. In a small bowl, whisk together the Bone Broth, arrowroot, salt, and pepper.

3. Pour the broth mixture over the vegetable mixture in the slow cooker, and add the chicken.

4. Cover and cook on low for 8 hours.

5. Stir in the parsley just before serving.

A LITTLE LESS PALEO: White wine pairs perfectly with tarragon. Replace 1 cup of chicken broth with the same amount of white wine.

PER SERVING CALORIES: 330; PROTEIN: 29G; CARBOHYDRATES: 24G; SUGAR: 12G; FAT: 15G; FIBER: 5G; SODIUM: 906MG

Chicken Cacciatore

PREP TIME: 20 MINUTES / COOK TIME: 8 HOURS

SERVES 6 Italian food prepared *alla cacciatora* means "hunter style." Chicken cacciatore, then, is a hunter-style stew featuring chicken and vegetables. This rich stew has sweet bell peppers, savory chicken, and plenty of fragrant garlic and herbs to fill you up after a long day.

1 onion, chopped

1 green bell pepper, seeded and chopped

1 red bell pepper, seeded and chopped

2 (14-ounce) cans crushed tomatoes, undrained

¼ cup capers, drained

1 tablespoon Italian seasoning

1 teaspoon garlic powder

1 teaspoon sea salt

¼ teaspoon freshly ground black pepper

Pinch red pepper flakes

¾ cup Bone Broth (page 26) made with chicken bones

1 tablespoon arrowroot powder

8 chicken thighs

¼ cup chopped fresh basil

1. In the slow cooker, combine the onion, bell peppers, tomatoes and their juice, capers, Italian seasoning, garlic powder, salt, pepper, and red pepper flakes.

2. In a small bowl, whisk together the Bone Broth and arrowroot. Stir the broth mixture in with the veggies in the slow cooker.

3. Place the chicken thighs in the slow cooker, pressing them into the vegetable mixture.

4. Cover and cook on low for 8 hours.

5. Stir in the basil just before serving.

A LITTLE LESS PALEO: Red wine is a flavorful addition to this stew. To use it, replace the broth with an equal amount of a dry red wine, such as Chianti.

PER SERVING CALORIES: 463; PROTEIN: 61G; CARBOHYDRATES: 17G; SUGAR: 10G; FAT: 16G; FIBER: 6G; SODIUM: 1,002MG

Mexican Chicken Stew

PREP TIME: 15 MINUTES / COOK TIME: 8 HOURS

SERVES 6 This savory stew is rich with chicken and spicy with peppers, and has plenty of satisfying vegetables. It's a delicious one-pot meal that will feed your entire family. You can make a double batch and freeze it, as it keeps well and makes great on-the-go meals when you're too busy to cook.

1½ pounds chicken thigh meat, cut into 1-inch pieces

1 pound pearl onions, peeled

2 green bell peppers, seeded and chopped

3 jalapeño peppers, seeded and chopped

4 large carrots, peeled and chopped

8 ounces cremini mushrooms, halved

1 (14-ounce) can crushed tomatoes, undrained

½ cup Bone Broth (page 26) made with chicken bones

Zest of 1 lime

1 tablespoon chili powder

1 teaspoon dried oregano

1 teaspoon ground cumin

1 teaspoon sea salt

½ teaspoon ground coriander

½ teaspoon chipotle chili powder

Juice of 1 lime

¼ cup chopped fresh cilantro

1. In the slow cooker, combine the chicken, onions, bell peppers, jalapeños, carrots, mushrooms, tomatoes and their juice, Bone Broth, lime zest, chili powder, oregano, cumin, salt, coriander, and chili powder.

2. Cover and cook on low for 8 hours.

3. Stir in the lime juice and cilantro just before serving.

A LITTLE LESS PALEO: Two tasty additions to this stew are 2 cups of fresh shelled peas (which are legumes and not technically Paleo) and a grating of Cotija cheese over the top.

PER SERVING CALORIES: 276; PROTEIN: 24G; CARBOHYDRATES: 24G; SUGAR: 12G; FAT: 11G; FIBER: 7G; SODIUM: 655MG

Chicken Mole

PREP TIME: 15 MINUTES / COOK TIME: 8 HOURS

SERVES 6 Mole is a traditional chocolate-based Mexican sauce that dates back to the sixteenth century. While we tend to think of chocolate as a sweet dessert, mole uses unsweetened cocoa and is quite savory. The warm, spicy sauce adds a deep, rich flavor to the chicken thigh meat and vegetables. Try serving it with cauliflower rice for a fully satisfying meal. Simply pulse cauliflower in a food processor or grate it and sauté in a little olive oil for about 5 minutes.

12 bone-in chicken thighs, skin removed

1 onion, chopped

1 (14-ounce) can crushed tomatoes, undrained

¼ cup dark cocoa powder

¼ cup almond butter

1 teaspoon chipotle chili powder

1 teaspoon chili powder

1 teaspoon garlic powder

1 teaspoon ground cumin

1 teaspoon sea salt

Dash ground cayenne pepper

1. In the slow cooker, combine the chicken thighs, onion, tomatoes and their juice, cocoa powder, almond butter, chili powders, garlic powder, cumin, salt, and cayenne, stirring to mix well.

2. Cover and cook on low for 8 hours, and serve.

> **PRECOOKING:** In a large pan over medium heat, brown the chicken thighs in 2 tablespoons of your favorite Paleo-friendly fat for 5 minutes per side before adding them to the slow cooker.

PER SERVING CALORIES: 271; PROTEIN: 31G; CARBOHYDRATES: 13G; SUGAR: 5G; FAT: 12G; FIBER: 5G; SODIUM: 588MG

Ground Turkey Lettuce Wraps

PREP TIME: 10 MINUTES / COOK TIME: 8 HOURS

QP

SERVES 6 This ground turkey recipe is golden and fragrant, thanks to the addition of turmeric. It gives the ground turkey an Asian flavor, especially with the addition of savory fish sauce, creamy almond butter, and zesty lime. You can make the turkey mixture ahead of time and reheat it, so it's a great take-to-work lunch.

1½ pounds ground turkey, crumbled

1 onion, chopped

1 cup Bone Broth (page 26) made with chicken bones

½ cup coconut milk

¼ cup almond butter

1 tablespoon honey

1 teaspoon Asian fish sauce

1 teaspoon ground turmeric

1 teaspoon garlic powder

1 teaspoon sea salt

½ teaspoon curry powder

Zest and juice of 1 lime

⅛ teaspoon freshly ground black pepper

¼ cup chopped fresh cilantro

12 large lettuce leaves

1. In the slow cooker, combine the turkey, onion, Bone Broth, coconut milk, almond butter, honey, fish sauce, turmeric, garlic powder, salt, curry powder, lime zest and juice, and pepper.

2. Cover and cook on low for 8 hours.

3. Stir in the cilantro before serving. To serve, spoon the turkey mixture onto the lettuce leaves to make wraps.

NUTRITION HIGHLIGHT: Turmeric has many health benefits, including as an anti-inflammatory and can potentially prevent certain cancers, according to World's Healthiest Foods. It has been used in traditional Chinese medicine for centuries.

PER SERVING CALORIES: 361; PROTEIN: 34G; CARBOHYDRATES: 9G; SUGAR: 5G; FAT: 23G; FIBER: 2G; SODIUM: 660MG

Basic Turkey Breast
WITH Root Vegetables

PREP TIME: 15 MINUTES / COOK TIME: 8 HOURS

SERVES 8 This turkey breast is simple and delicious. Flavored with fragrant herbs, the turkey juices drip down to the root vegetables, adding tremendous flavor. The turkey breast itself is usually pretty large (around 6 pounds), so this feeds a crowd or makes great leftovers. To store the cooked turkey breast, you can cut it into single-size portions and freeze it in zip-top bags.

8 ounces baby carrots

2 fennel bulbs, sliced

8 ounces pearl onions

8 ounces button mushrooms

1 teaspoon dried thyme

1 teaspoon dried rosemary

1 teaspoon sea salt

¼ teaspoon freshly ground black pepper

Zest of 1 lemon

1 whole turkey breast, skin on

1. In the bottom of the slow cooker, arrange the baby carrots, fennel, onions, and mushrooms.

2. In a small bowl, mix to combine the thyme, rosemary, salt, pepper, and lemon zest.

3. Rub the outside of the turkey breast with the salt mixture.

4. Place the turkey in the slow cooker on top of the vegetables.

5. Cover and cook on low for 8 hours, and serve.

PRECOOKING: You can add more flavor to the turkey breast by rubbing it with the salt mixture and letting it sit overnight, covered, in your refrigerator. This allows the seasoning to better penetrate the meat.

PER SERVING CALORIES: 347; PROTEIN: 60G; CARBOHYDRATES: 10G; SUGAR: 3G; FAT: 3G; FIBER: 4G; SODIUM: 814MG

Spinach-Stuffed Turkey Cutlets

PREP TIME: 15 MINUTES / COOK TIME: 8 HOURS

SERVES 6 These delicious and flavorful turkey cutlets have a pretty color and a bright herbal and citrus flavor. Purchase the turkey breast with the skin still on if you can. Remove the skin to make the cutlets, then wrap the skin around the cutlets to keep them moist while they cook, discarding the skin before serving the breast.

1 pound frozen spinach, thawed, excess water squeezed out

Zest of 1 orange

3 garlic cloves, chopped

2 cups almond meal

1 teaspoon dried thyme

Juice of 1 orange

2 teaspoons sea salt, divided

¼ teaspoon freshly ground black pepper, divided

2 pounds turkey breast meat, cut into 6 pieces and pounded into ¼-inch-thick cutlets

Turkey skin

2 cups Bone Broth (page 26) made with chicken bones

1. In a large bowl, mix the spinach, orange zest, garlic, almond meal, thyme, and orange juice with 1 teaspoon of salt and ⅛ teaspoon of pepper.

2. Season the turkey breast with the remaining 1 teaspoon of salt and ⅛ teaspoon of pepper.

3. Divide the spinach mixture into 6 portions, and spoon one portion atop each piece of turkey breast.

4. Roll the breast around the filling, and roll a piece of skin around the breast, tying with kitchen twine.

5. Place the stuffed breasts in the slow cooker, and add the Bone Broth. Cover and cook on low for 8 hours.

6. Remove and discard the skin and skim the fat before serving.

NUTRITION HIGHLIGHT: Almonds are an excellent source of biotin, which is a B complex vitamin that supports strong hair, nails, and connective tissue. They are also high in vitamin E, magnesium, and potassium.

PER SERVING CALORIES: 388; PROTEIN: 37G; CARBOHYDRATES: 21G; SUGAR: 10G; FAT: 19G; FIBER: 7G; SODIUM: 2,474MG

Turkey WITH Olives AND Mediterranean Spices

PREP TIME: 20 MINUTES / COOK TIME: 8 HOURS

SERVES 6 Olives add rich flavor to this turkey breast, while lemon adds acid and the Mediterranean spices offer savory flavors. As the recipe cooks, turkey juices drip on the eggplant, adding flavor to the vegetables, as well. If you find eggplant slightly bitter, you can salt slices of eggplant for 30 minutes, allowing the water to drip away through a colander, and then wipe away the salt with a piece of paper towel before cutting the eggplant into cubes and adding it to the slow cooker.

1½ pounds boneless, skinless turkey breast

2 cups Bone Broth (page 26) made with
    chicken bones

2 eggplants, cut into cubes

1 onion, chopped

8 ounces Kalamata olives, pitted and halved

Juice and zest of 1 lemon

1 teaspoon dried rosemary

1 teaspoon garlic powder

1 teaspoon ground cumin

1 teaspoon ground coriander

1 teaspoon dried oregano

½ teaspoon sea salt

¼ teaspoon ground cinnamon

1. In the slow cooker, combine the turkey, Bone Broth, eggplant, onion, olives, lemon juice and zest, rosemary, garlic powder, cumin, coriander, oregano, salt, and cinnamon.

2. Cover and cook on low for 8 hours, and serve.

NUTRITION HIGHLIGHT: Olives are high in antioxidants. They are also an excellent source of healthy monounsaturated fats.

PER SERVING CALORIES: 235; PROTEIN: 24G; CARBOHYDRATES: 22G; SUGAR: 11G; FAT: 7G; FIBER: 9G; SODIUM: 1,896MG

Duck Confit

PREP TIME: 15 MINUTES, PLUS 12 TO 24 HOURS TO MARINATE / COOK TIME: 8 HOURS

SERVES 6 Duck confit is a rich, savory dish of herbed duck legs cooked in duck fat. The result is unctuous and delicious, and it makes a tasty meal or snack by itself, with side dishes, on salads, or as some of the meat in other dishes. The slow cooker is the ideal device for making duck confit. You can find duck fat online, or check with your local butcher. Duck fat is expensive, but you can reuse it. After making the confit, strain the fat and save it in your refrigerator in a tightly sealed container for up to 6 months, or in your freezer for up to a year.

6 duck legs

½ cup sea salt

4 teaspoons dried thyme

3 bay leaves, crushed

1 tablespoon white pepper

2 teaspoons dried rosemary

7 cups duck fat

1. Pat the duck legs dry with a paper towel.

2. In a small bowl, mix the salt, thyme, bay leaves, white pepper, and rosemary.

3. Rub the spice mixture over the duck legs. Cover the duck legs and allow to sit for 12 to 24 hours in the refrigerator.

4. Rinse the legs and pat them dry.

5. Put the duck fat in the slow cooker, turn it to high, and melt the duck fat (or melt it in the microwave and add it to the slow cooker).

6. Add the legs, and turn the slow cooker down to low.

7. Cover and cook on low for 8 hours, and serve.

PORTION ADJUSTMENT: You can use fewer or more duck legs, depending on the size of your slow cooker. Just make sure the legs are completely covered with fat.

PER SERVING CALORIES: 310; PROTEIN: 31G; CARBOHYDRATES: 2G; SUGAR: 1G; FAT: 20G; FIBER: 0G; SODIUM: 1,140MG

Orange-Sriracha Duck Stew

PREP TIME: 15 MINUTES / COOK TIME: 8 HOURS

SERVES 6 Duck has a rich, meaty flavor that's delicious with citrus and sweeter fruits. Here, dried apricots and orange juice and zest cut through the richness, while spicy Orange-Chili-Garlic Sauce adds a hint of heat. This is a hearty meal that's perfect for cold nights in the winter or fall.

1 pound pearl onions, peeled

1½ pounds boneless, skinless duck breast, cut into 1-inch cubes

1 cup dried apricots

2 sweet potatoes, cubed

2 cups Bone Broth (page 26)

2 tablespoons arrowroot powder

1 tablespoon Orange-Chili-Garlic Sauce (page 28)

1 teaspoon garlic powder

Juice of 2 oranges

Zest of 1 orange

1 teaspoon sea salt

¼ teaspoon freshly ground black pepper

1. In the slow cooker, combine the onions, duck breast, dried apricots, and sweet potatoes.

2. In a small bowl, whisk together the Bone Broth, arrowroot, Orange-Chili-Garlic Sauce, garlic powder, orange juice and zest, salt, and pepper.

3. Pour the broth mixture over the duck in the slow cooker.

4. Cover and cook on low for 8 hours, and serve.

NUTRITION HIGHLIGHT: Apricots are high in beta-carotene, an antioxidant. They are also a good source of vitamin C and fiber.

PER SERVING CALORIES: 335; PROTEIN: 30G; CARBOHYDRATES: 42G; SUGAR: 12G; FAT: 6G; FIBER: 7G; SODIUM: 594MG

Duck WITH Fig Sauce

PREP TIME: 15 MINUTES / COOK TIME: 8 HOURS

SERVES 6 Figs and duck are a tasty flavor combination. The figs have a slight sweetness that pairs well with the richness of the duck. Figs are in season twice a year—in late spring and late summer/early fall—because fig trees produce fruit twice in a growing season. This recipe is best when figs are fresh in season.

1½ pounds boneless, skinless duck breast, cut into 1-inch cubes

1 onion, chopped

1 pound fresh figs, stems removed, halved

¼ cup balsamic vinegar

¼ cup honey

1 teaspoon garlic powder

2 cups Bone Broth (page 26)

2 tablespoons arrowroot powder

1 teaspoon dried thyme

1 teaspoon sea salt

¼ teaspoon freshly ground black pepper

Pinch red pepper flakes

1. In the slow cooker, combine the duck breast, onion, figs, vinegar, honey, and garlic powder.

2. In a small bowl, whisk together the Bone Broth, arrowroot, thyme, salt, pepper, and red pepper flakes.

3. Pour the broth mixture over the duck and figs in the slow cooker.

4. Cover and cook on low for 8 hours, and serve.

NUTRITION HIGHLIGHT: A member of the mulberry family, figs are filled with little seeds that add crunch and fiber to foods. Figs are also an excellent source of the mineral potassium.

PER SERVING CALORIES: 414; PROTEIN: 29G; CARBOHYDRATES: 65G; SUGAR: 49G; FAT: 6G; FIBER: 8G; SODIUM: 576MG

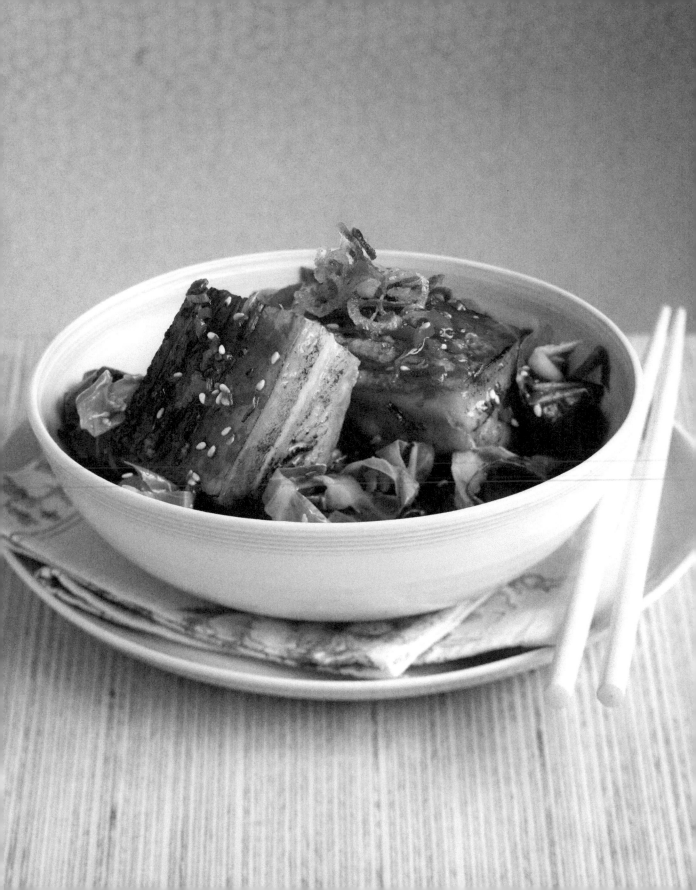

Italian Sausage AND Peppers

PREP TIME: 15 MINUTES / COOK TIME: 8 HOURS

SERVES 6 Combining onions, sausage, and peppers in one savory dish is an Italian tradition, and like most Italian foods, this meal is simply delicious. It is also a really easy recipe to scale up or down. Just plan on one to one and a half sausages per person, and about one pepper per person.

1½ pounds Italian sausage

1½ cups Bone Broth (page 26)

2 red bell peppers, seeded and sliced

2 green bell peppers, seeded and sliced

2 orange bell peppers, seeded and sliced

1 onion, chopped

¼ cup extra-virgin olive oil

1 teaspoon garlic powder

1 teaspoon dried oregano

1 teaspoon sea salt

¼ teaspoon freshly ground black pepper

Pinch red pepper flakes

1. Put the whole sausages and the Bone Broth in the slow cooker.

2. In a large bowl, toss the bell peppers, onion, olive oil, garlic powder, oregano, salt, pepper, and red pepper flakes to coat the peppers with the oil and spices.

3. Add the pepper mixture to the slow cooker.

4. Cover and cook on low for 8 hours, and serve.

A LITTLE LESS PALEO: This is a recipe that practically cries out for wine. Use a dry white wine, such as a Pinot Grigio or Chardonnay, and replace all the broth with an equal amount of the wine for an authentic Italian taste.

PER SERVING CALORIES: 508; PROTEIN: 24G; CARBOHYDRATES: 10G; SUGAR: 6G; FAT: 41G; FIBER: 3G; SODIUM: 1,202MG

Chorizo, Sweet Potato AND Chile Pepper Stew

PREP TIME: 15 MINUTES / COOK TIME: 8 HOURS

SERVES 6 Chorizo is a spicy, flavorful sausage originally from Spain and Portugal. It can be a bit hot, but the sweetness and the starch in the sweet potatoes soak up some of the heat of the chorizo. Chile peppers add freshness, and a dash of cilantro added at the end brings a nice fresh, herbal quality to the dish.

1½ pounds chorizo, sliced

4 cups cubed sweet potatoes

3 poblano peppers, seeded and minced

1 onion, chopped

1 teaspoon garlic powder

Juice of 1 orange

1 teaspoon sea salt

⅛ teaspoon freshly ground black pepper

¼ cup chopped fresh cilantro

Juice of 1 lime

1. In the slow cooker, combine the chorizo, sweet potatoes, peppers, onion, garlic powder, orange juice, salt, and pepper.

2. Cover and cook on low for 8 hours.

3. Stir in the cilantro and lime juice just before serving.

SEASONAL INGREDIENTS: In the winter, substitute the sweet potatoes with winter squash, such as acorn or butternut squash. You can also replace them with cubed pumpkin when it's available in the fall. The flavors and textures will be similar to the sweet potato.

PER SERVING CALORIES: 670; PROTEIN: 30G; CARBOHYDRATES: 39G; SUGAR: 6G; FAT: 44G; FIBER: 6G; SODIUM: 1,724MG

Linguica WITH Sweet Peppers AND Onions

PREP TIME: 15 MINUTES / COOK TIME: 8 HOURS

SERVES 6 Linguica, a flavorful Portuguese sausage, has mild heat and a lot of flavor. It's delicious with sweet bell peppers and onions, making a tasty, slightly smoky stew. Carrots and sweet potatoes make this a tasty one-pot meal that freezes and reheats well, so feel free to make a bigger batch.

1½ pounds linguica, sliced

1½ cups Bone Broth (page 26)

8 ounces baby carrots

2 cups cubed white sweet potatoes

2 red bell peppers, seeded and sliced

2 yellow bell peppers, seeded and sliced

2 orange bell peppers, seeded and sliced

1 red onion, sliced

1 teaspoon smoked paprika

1 teaspoon garlic powder

1 teaspoon sea salt

¼ teaspoon freshly ground black pepper

1. In the slow cooker, combine the linguica, Bone Broth, carrots, sweet potatoes, bell peppers, onion, paprika, garlic powder, salt, and pepper.

2. Cover and cook on low for 8 hours, and serve.

A LITTLE LESS PALEO: Potatoes are hotly debated in the Paleo community, but many Paleo dieters occasionally eat them. If you'd like to take a walk on the wild, slightly less Paleo, side, try replacing the white sweet potatoes with 2 cups of cubed purple potatoes. Update the flavor with a little wine as well, replacing the broth with an equal amount of a light red wine, such as Pinot Noir.

PER SERVING CALORIES: 487; PROTEIN: 22G; CARBOHYDRATES: 29G; SUGAR: 10G; FAT: 31G; FIBER: 6G; SODIUM: 1,338MG

Pork Carnitas Lettuce Wraps

PREP TIME: 15 MINUTES / COOK TIME: 8 HOURS

SERVES 8 Braised meat, carnitas, make the perfect taco filling in Mexican cuisine. Traditional carnitas are made from savory pork or beef with fragrant spices. These pork carnitas make the perfect filling for taco lettuce wraps, served with creamy chopped avocados and spicy Cooked Salsa (page 29).

2 pounds boneless pork shoulder, cut into 1-inch cubes

1 cup Bone Broth (page 26) made with beef bones

2 jalapeño peppers, seeded and minced

1 onion, chopped

1 teaspoon garlic powder

1 teaspoon chili powder

1 teaspoon ground cumin

1 teaspoon sea salt

¼ teaspoon freshly ground black pepper

16 large lettuce leaves

2 cups Cooked Salsa (page 29)

Two avocados, peeled, pitted, and cut into cubes

1. In the slow cooker, combine the pork shoulder, Bone Broth, jalapeños, onion, garlic powder, chili powder, cumin, salt, and pepper.

2. Cover and cook on low for 8 hours.

3. Serve the meat and veggies wrapped in the lettuce leaves, garnished with the Cooked Salsa and avocado.

NUTRITION HIGHLIGHT: Avocados are a very healthy Paleo food. Not only are they an excellent source of fiber (each avocado has 10 grams of fiber), but they are also rich in healthy monounsaturated fats and contain high levels of vitamins E, C, and K and folic acid.

PER SERVING CALORIES: 299; PROTEIN: 32G; CARBOHYDRATES: 12G; SUGAR: 4G; FAT: 14G; FIBER: 5G; SODIUM: 715MG

Honey Mustard–Pork Lettuce Wraps

PREP TIME: 20 MINUTES / COOK TIME: 8 HOURS

SERVES 8 The sweet honey and tangy mustard make these tender pork lettuce wraps really tasty. Pork shoulder, braised low and slow, shreds easily to make a nice filling. For a bit of crunchiness, you'll enjoy the tasty slaw that goes on top of the pork before you wrap it in the lettuce. The slaw is also a delicious topping for the Pulled Pork on page 152.

FOR THE PORK

2 pounds boneless pork shoulder

1 cup Bone Broth (page 26)

¼ cup honey

¼ cup Dijon mustard

1 teaspoon sea salt

¼ teaspoon freshly ground black pepper

16 large lettuce leaves

FOR THE SLAW

1 head cabbage, shredded

6 scallions, thinly sliced

¼ cup apple cider vinegar

Juice and zest of 1 orange

2 garlic cloves, finely minced

½ teaspoon sea salt

¼ teaspoon freshly ground black pepper

TO MAKE THE PORK

1. In the slow cooker, combine the pork shoulder, Bone Broth, honey, mustard, salt, and pepper.

2. Cover and cook on low for 8 hours.

3. Using 2 forks, shred the pork and mix with the sauce.

4. Wrap the pork in the lettuce leaves, topped with the slaw.

TO MAKE THE SLAW

1. In a large bowl, mix to combine the cabbage and scallions.

2. In a small bowl, whisk together the vinegar, orange juice and zest, garlic, salt, and pepper. Toss with the cabbage and scallions.

PRECOOKING: To add flavor, season the pork with the salt and pepper. Then heat 2 tablespoons of your favorite Paleo-friendly oil in a large sauté pan over medium heat. Sear the pork on all sides, about 5 minutes per side, before adding it to the slow cooker. Deglaze the pan with the broth, using a wooden spoon to scrape any browned bits from the bottom of the pan. Pour the liquid into the slow cooker with the pork, adding the mustard and honey. Cover and cook on low for 8 hours.

PER SERVING CALORIES: 248; PROTEIN: 33G; CARBOHYDRATES: 20G; SUGAR: 15G; FAT: 5G; FIBER: 4G; SODIUM: 560MG

Ground Pork Stew

PREP TIME: 20 MINUTES / COOK TIME: 8 HOURS

SERVES 6 Ground pork is a very versatile meat. It has a lighter flavor than ground beef, and won't overwhelm a dish. Here, it pairs well with the spices and flavorful vegetables. If you want to save time, replace the fresh pearl onions with frozen ones, which are already peeled and therefore much easier to add to this stew.

1½ pounds ground pork

1 pound cremini mushrooms, quartered

8 ounces pearl onions, peeled

2 carrots, peeled and sliced

1 green bell pepper

1 teaspoon ground cumin

1 teaspoon ground coriander

1 teaspoon chili powder

1 teaspoon garlic powder

Dash ground cayenne pepper

2 (14-ounce) cans tomato sauce

1 teaspoon sea salt

1. In the slow cooker, crumble the ground pork. Add the mushrooms, onion, carrots, bell pepper, cumin, coriander, chili powder, garlic powder, cayenne, tomato sauce, and salt.

2. Cover and cook on low for 8 hours, and serve.

MAKE-AHEAD TIP: To give a deeper flavor, brown the ground pork before adding it to the slow cooker. Heat a large sauté pan over medium-high heat, adding 1 tablespoon of your favorite Paleo-friendly oil. Crumble the pork and cook, stirring occasionally, until browned, about 5 minutes.

PER SERVING CALORIES: 247; PROTEIN: 34G; CARBOHYDRATES: 18G; SUGAR: 10G; FAT: 5G; FIBER: 5G; SODIUM: 1,100MG

Salsa Pork Shoulder

PREP TIME: 5 MINUTES / COOK TIME: 8 HOURS

SERVES 6 It doesn't get any easier than this spicy salsa pork. Eat it like a bowl of chili, or serve with chopped avocados and sliced scallions as garnish. You can even wrap it in lettuce leaves to make tacos. This dish also freezes well. Make the salsa ahead of time, or find a Paleo brand you like if you don't feel like making the salsa yourself.

2 pounds pork shoulder, cut into 1-inch cubes

1 onion, chopped

2 cups Cooked Salsa (page 29)

½ teaspoon sea salt

1. In the slow cooker, combine the pork shoulder, onion, Cooked Salsa, and salt.

2. Cover and cook on low for 8 hours, and serve.

NUTRITION HIGHLIGHT: Salsa is a really healthy condiment. With tomatoes that are packed with antioxidants like lycopene, chiles that are another good source of lycopene, and plenty of vitamins and minerals, salsa is a healthy way to add flavor and spice up many Paleo dishes. Trader Joe's salsa is a healthy Paleo brand that is worth a try.

PER SERVING CALORIES: 472; PROTEIN: 37G; CARBOHYDRATES: 7G; SUGAR: 3G; FAT: 33G; FIBER: 2G; SODIUM: 780MG

Pork Meatballs WITH Mushroom Gravy

PREP TIME: 20 MINUTES / COOK TIME: 8 HOURS

SERVES 6 Thyme-scented meatballs cooked in a rich mushroom broth make for a hearty meal. Try them with some Roasted Garlic Cauliflower Mash (page 55), which soaks up the gravy and takes on its rich, earthy flavors. Almond meal replaces breadcrumbs in the meatballs, keeping everything Paleo and giving them a lighter, less dense texture.

1½ pounds ground pork

2 carrots, peeled and grated

1 tablespoon Dijon mustard

2 teaspoons dried thyme, divided

1 teaspoon Asian fish sauce

1 teaspoon garlic powder

1 teaspoon onion powder

1 cup almond meal

2 eggs, beaten

2 teaspoons sea salt, divided

¼ teaspoon freshly ground black pepper, divided

4 cups Mushroom Stock (page 23)

8 ounces mushrooms, sliced

8 ounces baby carrots

1 onion, chopped

6 garlic cloves, halved

1. In a large bowl, mix the ground pork, carrots, mustard, 1 teaspoon of thyme, fish sauce, garlic powder, onion powder, almond meal, eggs, 1 teaspoon of salt, and ⅛ teaspoon of pepper.

2. Roll the meat into 1-inch meatballs, and put them in the slow cooker.

3. Add the Mushroom Stock, mushrooms, carrots, onion, garlic, and the remaining 1 teaspoon of thyme, 1 teaspoon of salt, and ⅛ teaspoon of pepper.

4. Cover and cook on low for 8 hours.

5. Using a slotted spoon, lift out the meatballs and set them aside on a platter.

6. Using a potato masher, mash the carrots and vegetables, or purée in a blender or food processor, until the liquid is thick and gravy-like.

7. Serve the meatballs topped with the gravy.

NUTRITION HIGHLIGHT: Not all fish sauce is created equal—and not all of it is Paleo, because it may contain sugar or other ingredients besides fish and salt. Fortunately, there are some Paleo brands made only from fermented fish and sea salt that you can use, such as Red Boat, made from anchovies, sea salt, and nothing else.

PER SERVING CALORIES: 348; PROTEIN: 40G; CARBOHYDRATES: 14G; SUGAR: 6G; FAT: 15G; FIBER: 5G; SODIUM: 1,372MG

Pulled Pork

PREP TIME: 15 MINUTES / COOK TIME: 8 HOURS

SERVES 8 If you're craving Southern barbecue, pulled pork is the dish for you! Pork shoulder lends itself perfectly to pulled pork because it cooks best low and slow, so that the fat has time to render, and the collagen melts and softens. Many people use pulled pork as a tasty and tangy sandwich filling. Here, you can serve it on top of a healthy salad or make a wrap out of it with thick lettuce leaves. Some people even enjoy using grilled Portobello mushrooms as a sandwich wrap for pulled pork. The slaw for the Honey Mustard–Pork Lettuce Wraps (page 146) pairs well with this dish.

2 pounds boneless pork shoulder

1 (4-ounce) can tomato paste

1 (14-ounce) can tomato sauce

½ cup apple cider vinegar

¼ cup pure maple syrup

1 teaspoon chipotle chili powder

1 teaspoon garlic powder

1 teaspoon onion powder

1 teaspoon sea salt

½ teaspoon liquid smoke

¼ teaspoon freshly ground black pepper

1. In the slow cooker, combine the pork shoulder, tomato paste and sauce, vinegar, syrup, chili powder, garlic powder, onion powder, salt, liquid smoke, and pepper.

2. Cover and cook on low for 8 hours.

3. Using 2 forks, shred the pork shoulder. Mix the meat with the sauce, and serve.

PORTION ADJUSTMENT: This is a really easy recipe to size up or down, depending on the size of your slow cooker. It's an especially easy recipe to make for a large crowd. To make portion adjustments, keep the same amount of sauce ingredients and just add larger or smaller pieces of pork. Cut the pork into two or three pieces if needed so it fits in the slow cooker.

PER SERVING CALORIES: 218; PROTEIN: 31G; CARBOHYDRATES: 13G; SUGAR: 10G; FAT: 4G; FIBER: 2G; SODIUM: 578MG

Pork Shoulder WITH Apples, Fennel, AND Cabbage

PREP TIME: 15 MINUTES / COOK TIME: 8 HOURS

SERVES 6 This tasty, hearty dish is a combination of savory and sweet. The apples add a sweet-tart flavor, while the fennel, cabbage, and pork add savory tastes perfectly complemented by the herbs and spices in the dish. Choose a variety of sweet-tart apple, such as Braeburn or Honeycrisp, for this dish.

2 pounds pork shoulder, cut into 1-inch cubes

2 apples, peeled, cored, and sliced

1 fennel bulb, sliced

1 head cabbage, shredded

1 red onion, sliced

1 teaspoon dried thyme

¼ cup apple cider vinegar

1 tablespoon Dijon mustard

1 teaspoon garlic powder

1 teaspoon sea salt

⅛ teaspoon freshly ground black pepper

1. In the slow cooker, combine the pork shoulder, apples, fennel bulb, cabbage, red onion, thyme, vinegar, mustard, garlic powder, salt, and pepper.

2. Cover and cook on low for 8 hours, and serve.

PRECOOKING: To add deeper flavors, you can brown the pork shoulder before adding it to the slow cooker. Heat a large sauté pan over medium-high heat, adding 2 tablespoons of your favorite Paleo-friendly oil. Working in batches so you don't overcrowd the pan, cook the cubes until browned on all sides, 3 to 5 minutes per side.

PER SERVING CALORIES: 528; PROTEIN: 38G; CARBOHYDRATES: 21G; SUGAR: 11G; FAT: 33G; FIBER: 6G; SODIUM: 488MG

Maple Chipotle–Glazed Pork Shoulder

PREP TIME: 10 MINUTES / COOK TIME: 8 HOURS

SERVES 12 The combination of sweet and spicy is a classic one—the heat tones down the sweetness, and vice versa. Here, chipotle also adds a nice bit of smoke, while maple adds richness to the earthy flavor of the pork. Pork shoulder is so fatty that it doesn't need much liquid to braise, so this dish comes together quickly and easily. For a simple meal, serve it with a side salad.

2 pounds pork shoulder, cut into 1-inch cubes

½ cup pure maple syrup

Juice and zest of 1 orange

1 teaspoon chipotle chili powder

1 teaspoon garlic powder

1 teaspoon onion powder

1 teaspoon sea salt

¼ teaspoon freshly ground black pepper

1. Put the pork shoulder in the slow cooker.

2. In a small bowl, whisk together the maple syrup, orange juice and zest, chili powder, garlic powder, onion powder, salt, and pepper.

3. Pour the mixture over the pork.

4. Cover and cook on low for 8 hours, and serve.

SEASONAL INGREDIENTS: This recipe is delicious with apples or pears when they are in season. Peel and core three apples or pears. Slice them and add them to the slow cooker with the pork.

PER SERVING CALORIES: 529; PROTEIN: 36G; CARBOHYDRATES: 22G; SUGAR: 19G; FAT: 33G; FIBER: 1G; SODIUM: 422MG

Jalapeño AND Honey Pork Shoulder

PREP TIME: 10 MINUTES / COOK TIME: 8 HOURS

SERVES 6 The sweetness of honey blends beautifully with the heat of jalapeño peppers. You can adjust the number of jalapeños to make this dish spicier or milder. Including the seeds will add even more heat, so keep them if you dare. Serve with a side salad for a balanced meal.

2 pounds pork shoulder, cut into 1-inch cubes

¼ cup honey

Juice and zest of 1 orange

4 jalapeño peppers, seeded and minced

1 teaspoon garlic powder

1 teaspoon sea salt

⅛ teaspoon freshly ground black pepper

Dash ground cayenne pepper

1. In the slow cooker, combine the pork shoulder, honey, orange juice and zest, jalapeños, garlic powder, salt, pepper, and cayenne.

2. Cover and cook on low for 8 hours, and serve.

PRECOOKING: To add deeper flavor, brown the pork before adding it to the slow cooker. Melt 2 tablespoons of coconut oil in a large sauté pan over medium-high heat. Working in batches, brown the pork cubes, about 5 minutes per side. Don't overcrowd the pan, or you'll wind up steaming the pork and not getting the browned bits on the outside that add the deeper flavors.

PER SERVING CALORIES: 503; PROTEIN: 36G; CARBOHYDRATES: 16G; SUGAR: 15G; FAT: 33G; FIBER: 1G; SODIUM: 416MG

Pork AND Pineapple Teriyaki

PREP TIME: 10 MINUTES / COOK TIME: 8 HOURS

SERVES 12 If you like the sweet, tangy, slightly salty and spicy flavor of teriyaki, then you'll love this pork. What you'll like even more is just how easy it is to make this traditional Japanese dish. Chunks of pineapple and broccoli make this a tasty one-dish meal. If you want, try serving it with a little riced cauliflower. Simply pulse cauliflower in a food processor or grate it and sauté in a little olive oil for about 5 minutes.

2 pounds pork shoulder, cut into 1-inch cubes

1 pound broccoli, cut into florets

2 cups fresh pineapple, cut into chunks

½ cup coconut aminos

Juice of 1 orange

3 tablespoons honey

2 tablespoons arrowroot powder

1 tablespoon Orange-Chili-Garlic Sauce (page 28)

1 tablespoon grated fresh ginger

1 teaspoon garlic powder

2 tablespoons sesame seeds

3 scallions, thinly sliced on an angle

1. In the slow cooker, combine the pork shoulder, broccoli, and pineapple.

2. In a small bowl, whisk together the coconut aminos, orange juice, honey, arrowroot, Orange-Chili-Garlic Sauce, ginger, and garlic powder. Pour the sauce mixture over the pork and veggies in the slow cooker.

3. Cover and cook on low for 8 hours.

4. Sprinkle with the sesame seeds and scallions just before serving.

NUTRITION HIGHLIGHTS: Sesame seeds add a nutty flavor and a little bit of texture to this dish. They're also nutritional powerhouses, so if you like them, feel free to add a few more. The seeds are high in fiber and contain copper, calcium, magnesium, manganese, iron, and zinc—all minerals your body needs for good health.

PER SERVING CALORIES: 599; PROTEIN: 39G; CARBOHYDRATES: 34G; SUGAR: 19G; FAT: 34G; FIBER: 4G; SODIUM: 171MG

Dry-Rubbed Pork Ribs

PREP TIME: 10 MINUTES / COOK TIME: 8 HOURS

SERVES 6 The weather isn't always right for outdoor barbecuing, but thanks to your slow cooker, you can have the smoky, savory flavor of barbecued pork ribs even in the dead of winter. The dry rub seasons the ribs beautifully, and the moist environment of the slow cooker leaves them fall-off-the-bone-tender.

1½ teaspoons sea salt

¼ cup coconut sugar

1 tablespoon chili powder

1 tablespoon ground smoked paprika

1 teaspoon ground cumin

1 teaspoon garlic powder

1 teaspoon onion powder

1 teaspoon dried oregano

½ teaspoon freshly ground black pepper

2 racks pork loin back ribs
    (about 4 pounds total)

1. In a small bowl, mix to combine the salt, coconut sugar, chili powder, paprika, cumin, garlic powder, onion powder, oregano, and pepper.

2. Cut each rack of ribs into three pieces, and pat the ribs dry with a paper towel. Rub the spice mixture evenly over the ribs, and put them in the slow cooker.

3. Cover and cook on low for 8 hours, and serve.

> **PRECOOKING:** To really allow the rub to penetrate the meat, rub the spices on the night before. Wrap the rubbed ribs in foil and refrigerate for 12 hours, or overnight, before putting them in the slow cooker.

PER SERVING CALORIES: 662; PROTEIN: 61G; CARBOHYDRATES: 10G; SUGAR: 9G; FAT: 41G; FIBER: 1G; SODIUM: 614MG

Orange-Chipotle Country-Style Ribs

PREP TIME: 10 MINUTES / COOK TIME: 8 HOURS

SERVES 6 A little sweet and a little smoky heat makes these ribs flavorful and aromatic. Adding carrots makes it a one-pot meal that's quick and convenient. These ribs freeze well, so you can make big batches and enjoy them later, when you don't feel like cooking, but thawing and reheating seems easy.

2 pounds boneless country-style spare ribs

1 pound baby carrots

1 onion, chopped

1 cup Bone Broth (page 26)

Juice of 2 oranges

2 tablespoons honey

1 teaspoon garlic powder

1 teaspoon chipotle chili powder

1 teaspoon sea salt

¼ teaspoon freshly ground black pepper

1. In the slow cooker, combine the ribs, carrots, onion, Bone Broth, orange juice, honey, garlic powder, chili powder, salt, and pepper.

2. Cover and cook on low for 8 hours, and serve.

A LITTLE LESS PALEO: For a richer flavor, replace the broth with an equal amount of a sweet white wine, such as Riesling.

PER SERVING CALORIES: 387; PROTEIN: 32G; CARBOHYDRATES: 22G; SUGAR: 16G; FAT: 19G; FIBER: 4G; SODIUM: 523MG

Sweet AND Sour Country-Style Ribs

PREP TIME: 10 MINUTES / COOK TIME: 8 HOURS

SERVES 6 The glaze has a mouth-watering sweet and sour flavor, a perfect balance between the two flavors, with a bit of savory thrown in as well. They lend themselves well to slow cooking due to their high fat content and come out moist and tender. Serve with steamed vegetables for a complete meal.

2 pounds country-style spare ribs

1 cup unsweetened pineapple juice

¼ cup coconut aminos

¼ cup apple cider vinegar

1 tablespoon Orange-Chili-Garlic
   Sauce (page 28)

1 tablespoon arrowroot powder

1 teaspoon Asian fish sauce

1 teaspoon garlic powder

1 teaspoon onion powder

½ teaspoon sea salt

1. Arrange the ribs in the slow cooker.

2. In a medium bowl, whisk together the pineapple juice, coconut aminos, vinegar, Orange-Chili-Garlic Sauce, arrowroot, fish sauce, garlic powder, onion powder, and salt.

3. Pour the sauce over the pork.

4. Cover and cook on low for 8 hours, and serve.

PRECOOKING: To add deeper flavor, brown the pork before adding it to the slow cooker. Melt 2 tablespoons of coconut oil in a large sauté pan over medium-high heat. Working in batches, brown the ribs, about 5 minutes per side.

PER SERVING CALORIES: 262; PROTEIN: 29G; CARBOHYDRATES: 10G; SUGAR: 5G; FAT: 11G; FIBER: 0G; SODIUM: 736MG

Kalua Pork Roast

PREP TIME: 10 MINUTES / COOK TIME: 16 HOURS

QP

SERVES 12 In Hawaii, they cook pork underground with smoldering heat until it is very tender—a technique called "kalua." While you may not be able to bury a pig in your backyard to cook it, you can certainly cook pork in the slow cooker low and slow to create this tender and flavorful traditional Hawaiian dish. This recipe uses a lot of pork, so feel free to halve the recipe by cutting the roast in half and freezing half of it for another use. Alternatively, you can freeze the cooked meat in zip-top bags for reheating.

1 (5- to 6-pound) pork butt roast

1 tablespoon liquid smoke

1 tablespoon sea salt

1. Prick holes in the pork roast using a sharp knife or fork.

2. Rub the liquid smoke and salt all over the roast, and put it in the slow cooker.

3. Cover and cook on low for 16 hours.

PORTION ADJUSTMENT: You can easily make more or less by cutting the roast in half or quarters to make smaller or larger pieces and reducing the amount of liquid smoke and salt accordingly. It won't take as long with a smaller roast: For quarters, plan on 8 hours; for halves, plan on about 12.

PER SERVING CALORIES: 438; PROTEIN: 71G; CARBOHYDRATES: 0G; SUGAR: 0G; FAT: 15G; FIBER: 0G; SODIUM: 595MG

Mustard AND Herb Pork Loin

PREP TIME: 10 MINUTES / COOK TIME: 8 HOURS

SERVES 8 Mustard, rosemary, thyme, and garlic enhance the savory and mild flavor of a pork loin. Boneless pork loin can weigh anywhere up to 10 pounds. You can either cook the whole thing, or cut the loin into smaller portions, freezing the rest and just cooking what you need.

1 pound baby carrots

4 cups peeled and cubed celeriac

¼ cup chopped fresh parsley

3 tablespoons Dijon mustard

2 tablespoons extra-virgin olive oil

2 teaspoons dried thyme

2 teaspoons dried rosemary

1½ teaspoons sea salt

½ teaspoon freshly ground black pepper

1 (4-pound) boneless pork loin

1. In the slow cooker, combine the baby carrots and celeriac.

2. In a small bowl, whisk together the parsley, mustard, olive oil, thyme, rosemary, salt, and pepper.

3. Rub the mustard and herb mixture all over the outside of the pork loin. Arrange the loin in the slow cooker on top of the vegetables.

4. Cover and cook on low for 8 hours, and serve.

NUTRITION HIGHLIGHT: Rosemary is a fragrant herb that also has health benefits, according to World's Healthiest Foods. For example, rosemary has immune-boosting properties and anti-inflammatory compounds. It may also help improve circulation.

PER SERVING CALORIES: 414; PROTEIN: 61G; CARBOHYDRATES: 13G; SUGAR: 4G; FAT: 12G; FIBER: 4G; SODIUM: 670MG

Thai Pork Loaf

PREP TIME: 20 MINUTES / COOK TIME: 8 HOURS

SERVES 6 This meatloaf has spicy and savory Thai flavors that make it addicting. Lots of grated veggies lighten up the loaf and add plenty of nutritional value. You can eat the loaf by itself, since it's packed with vegetables, or serve it alongside Roasted Garlic Cauliflower Mash (page 55) or Sweet Potato Mash (page 50).

Paleo-friendly fat or oil, for greasing

1½ pounds ground pork

8 ounces shiitake mushrooms, finely chopped

1 onion, grated

3 stalks lemongrass, finely chopped

3 carrots, peeled and grated

2 cups grated cabbage

1 egg, beaten

2 tablespoons coconut aminos

1 tablespoon honey

1 tablespoon Orange-Chili-Garlic Sauce (page 28)

1 teaspoon Asian fish sauce

1 teaspoon garlic powder

1 teaspoon sea salt

¼ teaspoon freshly ground black pepper

1. Using your favorite Paleo-friendly fat or oil, grease the slow cooker insert.

2. In a large bowl, mix together the ground pork, mushrooms, onion, lemongrass, carrots, cabbage, egg, coconut aminos, honey, Orange-Chili-Garlic Sauce, fish sauce, garlic powder, salt, and pepper.

3. In the bottom of the slow cooker, form the mixture into a loaf.

4. Cover and cook on low for 8 hours, and serve.

A LITTLE LESS PALEO: Soy sauce, Worcestershire sauce, and sriracha are all delicious non-Paleo additions to this meatloaf. If you use soy sauce, eliminate the coconut aminos and be sure to get gluten-free soy sauce. Worcestershire sauce can replace the fish sauce in equal amounts. Sriracha can replace Orange-Chili-Garlic Sauce in an equal amount, or to taste.

PER SERVING CALORIES: 240; PROTEIN: 32G; CARBOHYDRATES: 16G; SUGAR: 7G; FAT: 5G; FIBER: 3G; SODIUM: 604MG

Asian Pear–Ginger Pork Belly

PREP TIME: 20 MINUTES / COOK TIME: 8 HOURS

SERVES 6 Pork belly is really just bacon that hasn't been cured, smoked, or sliced. It's also incredibly delicious, even when it isn't bacon. Check with your butcher or local farmers' market for pork belly, or you can find it online. Tenderbelly (see Resources) is an excellent, affordable source of naturally raised, pastured Berkshire pork belly.

2 pounds pork belly, sliced into ¼-inch-thick pieces

4 Asian pears, peeled, cored, and sliced

¼ cup coconut aminos

2 tablespoons Orange-Chili-Garlic Sauce (page 28)

2 tablespoons arrowroot powder

1 tablespoon grated fresh ginger

4 garlic cloves, minced

Juice of 1 orange

3 tablespoons sesame seeds

3 scallions, thinly sliced on an angle

1. In the bottom of the slow cooker, arrange the pork belly and Asian pears.

2. In a small bowl, whisk together the coconut aminos, Orange-Chili-Garlic Sauce, arrowroot, ginger, garlic, and orange juice. Pour the sauce mixture over the pork belly.

3. Cover and cook on low for 8 hours.

4. Sprinkle with the sesame seeds and scallions just before serving.

PRECOOKING: You can add flavor by browning the pork belly ahead of time. Brown it for 3 minutes per side in a large sauté pan over medium-high heat (no added fat is necessary). Add it to the slow cooker, reserving the fat in the pan (which is lard) for a later use. To save the lard, refrigerate it in a tightly sealed container.

PER SERVING CALORIES: 844; PROTEIN: 72G; CARBOHYDRATES: 31G; SUGAR: 17G; FAT: 43G; FIBER: 6G; SODIUM: 2,493MG

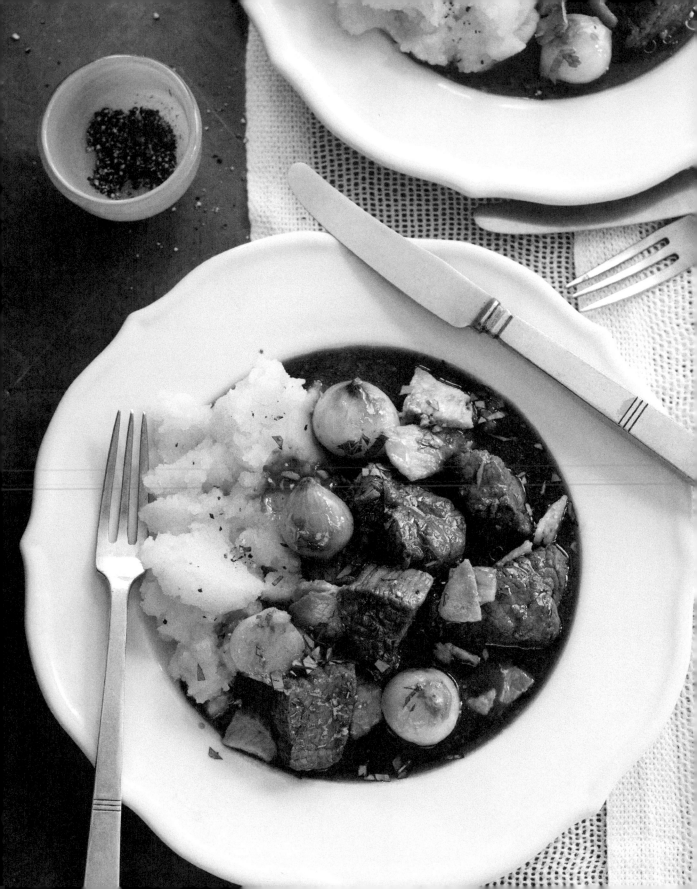

Beef and Lamb

Sloppy Joe Lettuce Cups

PREP TIME: 20 MINUTES / COOK TIME: 8 HOURS

SERVES 6 Sloppy Joes are an American classic. They're a family weeknight meal favorite, but they often come from a can and spill over the sides of a hamburger bun. This recipe keeps all the flavors of sloppy Joes, but lightens them up and makes them completely Paleo. The recipe freezes well, and it's also easy to double or triple for large groups—or leftovers.

2 pounds ground beef

2 green bell peppers, seeded and chopped

2 red bell peppers, seeded and chopped

1 onion, chopped

¼ cup apple cider vinegar

2 (14-ounce) cans crushed tomatoes

1 tablespoon chili powder

1 teaspoon garlic powder

1 teaspoon ground smoked paprika

1 teaspoon sea salt

¼ teaspoon freshly ground black pepper

Dash ground cayenne pepper

1 head iceberg lettuce, cut into 6 wedges, with the centers removed to form 6 cups

1. In the slow cooker, crumble the ground beef. Add the bell peppers, onion, vinegar, crushed tomatoes, chili powder, garlic powder, paprika, salt, pepper, and cayenne.

2. Cover and cook on low for 8 hours.

3. Spoon the sloppy Joe mixture into the lettuce cups and serve.

A LITTLE LESS PALEO: Make an adult version of sloppy Joes by adding whiskey or gluten-free beer in place of the apple cider vinegar. Use an equal amount (¼ cup).

PER SERVING CALORIES: 382; PROTEIN: 51G; CARBOHYDRATES: 20G; SUGAR: 12G; FAT: 10G; FIBER: 7G; SODIUM: 686MG

Beef Tacos

PREP TIME: 15 MINUTES / COOK TIME: 8 HOURS

SERVES 6 Flank steak has a deep flavor that makes it delicious for beef tacos. In this simple recipe, you combine strips of flank steak with a tasty marinade, then serve it wrapped in lettuce and topped with salsa and avocado slices. To ensure the flank steak is tender, when you cut it into strips, cut against the grain. To save time when making the marinade, pulse all the ingredients in a food processor or blender.

Juice of 3 limes

¼ cup avocado oil

2 jalapeño peppers, seeded and finely minced

6 scallions, very finely minced

6 garlic cloves, finely minced

¼ cup finely chopped cilantro

1 teaspoon ground cumin

1 teaspoon sea salt

¼ teaspoon freshly ground black pepper

Dash ground cayenne pepper

2 pounds flank steak, cut into 1-inch strips

12 lettuce leaves

2 avocados, cubed

2 cups Cooked Salsa (page 29)

1. In a small bowl, whisk together the lime juice, avocado oil, jalapeños, scallions, garlic, cilantro, cumin, salt, black pepper, and cayenne.

2. In the slow cooker, toss the marinade with the steak.

3. Cover and cook on low for 8 hours.

4. Serve the steak in the lettuce leaves topped with the avocados and Cooked Salsa.

PRECOOKING: Marinate the steak in a zip-top bag overnight before adding it to the slow cooker. This really allows the flavors of the marinade to penetrate the meat before it cooks.

PER SERVING CALORIES: 421; PROTEIN: 45G; CARBOHYDRATES: 13G; SUGAR: 4G; FAT: 21G; FIBER: 6G; SODIUM: 1,047MG

Classic Meatloaf

PREP TIME: 20 MINUTES / COOK TIME: 8 HOURS

SERVES 8 This is the meatloaf your mom used to make, although she probably made it in the oven, not the slow cooker. Still, it's rich with the memories, of childhood, and topped with a tangy tomato and maple glaze. If you were like most kids, you probably had your meatloaf with mashed potatoes. Try them with either the Roasted Garlic Cauliflower Mash (page 55), or the Sweet Potato Mash (page 50) for a meal that will take you back to your childhood.

Paleo-friendly fat or oil, for greasing

1 pound ground beef

½ pound ground pork

½ pound ground veal

1 cup almond meal

½ cup unsweetened almond milk

1 onion, chopped

2 tablespoons Dijon mustard

2 tablespoons coconut aminos

1 tablespoon fresh grated horseradish

1 teaspoon dried thyme

1 teaspoon garlic powder

1 teaspoon sea salt

¼ teaspoon freshly ground black pepper

¼ cup tomato paste

¼ cup apple cider vinegar

¼ cup pure maple syrup

Dash ground cayenne pepper

1. Using your favorite Paleo-friendly fat or oil, grease the slow cooker insert.

2. In a large bowl, mix to combine the beef, pork, veal, almond meal, almond milk, onion, mustard, coconut aminos, horseradish, thyme, garlic powder, salt, and pepper.

3. In the bottom of the slow cooker, form the meat mixture into a loaf.

4. In a small bowl, whisk together the tomato paste, vinegar, syrup, and cayenne.

5. Spread the sauce mixture over the meatloaf.

6. Cover and cook on low for 8 hours, and serve.

NUTRITION HIGHLIGHT:
Horseradish is actually a root vegetable, related to other types of radishes, but it is most frequently used as a spice because of its heat. According to *Life Extension Magazine*, horseradish has numerous health properties, including defending against certain cancers and immune-boosting properties. This is most likely due to the presence of compounds called "glucosinolates," which are also present in mustard.

PER SERVING CALORIES: 314; PROTEIN: 35G; CARBOHYDRATES: 14G; SUGAR: 8G; FAT: 13G; FIBER: 3G; SODIUM: 387MG

Ground Beef–Stuffed Peppers

PREP TIME: 20 MINUTES / COOK TIME: 8 HOURS

SERVES 4 Stuffed peppers are another American classic. The red bell peppers add sweetness to the savory filling. Almond meal lightens up the ground beef a bit, as do lots of chopped or grated vegetables. These stuffed peppers travel and reheat well, so they're excellent for making ahead and taking when you need something portable.

1 pound ground beef

2 carrots, peeled and grated

8 ounces cremini mushrooms, finely chopped

2 zucchini, grated

1 onion, chopped

½ cup almond meal

1 egg, beaten

1 tablespoon Dijon mustard

1 teaspoon garlic powder

1 teaspoon dried thyme

1 teaspoon sea salt

1 teaspoon coconut aminos

½ teaspoon Asian fish sauce

¼ teaspoon freshly ground black pepper

4 red bell peppers, tops, seeds, and ribs removed

1. In a large bowl, use your hands to mix the ground beef, carrots, mushrooms, zucchini, onion, almond meal, egg, mustard, garlic powder, thyme, salt, coconut aminos, fish sauce, and pepper until well combined.

2. Divide the mixture evenly among the 4 prepared peppers. Place the peppers, cut-side up, in the slow cooker.

3. Cover and cook on low for 8 hours, and serve.

NUTRITION HIGHLIGHT: Bell peppers are nightshade vegetables. Green, yellow, red, and orange bell peppers are all the same species, and they have similar nutritional qualities, so you can use them interchangeably. All are a great source of antioxidants, and contain capsaicin.

PER SERVING CALORIES: 314; PROTEIN: 35G; CARBOHYDRATES: 14G; SUGAR: 8G; FAT: 13G; FIBER: 3G; SODIUM: 387MG

Mushroom-Braised Brisket

PREP TIME: 20 MINUTES / COOK TIME: 8 HOURS

SERVES 8 Brisket is a cut of beef that lends itself well to slow cooking because it has a lot of intramuscular fat and tougher meat which gets very tender in a low, temperature, moist environment. The result is a tender, flavorful cut of meat seasoned with earthy mushrooms and herbs.

3 pounds brisket

1 pound cremini mushrooms, sliced

2 onions, sliced

1½ cups Mushroom Stock (page 23)

2 tablespoons coconut aminos

1 teaspoon garlic powder

1 teaspoon sea salt

¼ teaspoon freshly ground black pepper

1. In the slow cooker, mix to combine the brisket, mushrooms, onions, Mushroom Stock, coconut aminos, garlic powder, salt, and pepper.

2. Cover and cook on low for 8 hours, and serve.

A LITTLE LESS PALEO: If you've never had "drunken beef brisket" before, you'll discover this is definitely a worthy reason to be a little less Paleo. Drunken brisket is flavored with whiskey, and it's delicious. To make it, replace ½ cup of the broth with the same amount of whiskey and add 1 teaspoon of liquid smoke. Chop some scallions, and scatter them over the finished product for a little extra flavor.

PER SERVING CALORIES: 516; PROTEIN: 79G; CARBOHYDRATES: 8G; SUGAR: 3G; FAT: 16G; FIBER: 1G; SODIUM: 637MG

Pot Roast WITH Root Vegetables AND Mushrooms

PREP TIME: 15 MINUTES / COOK TIME: 8 HOURS

SERVES 8 Pot roast is an American classic, and making it in a slow cooker helps transform what is usually a tough cut of meat into very tender. This easy version includes root veggies, mushrooms, and fragrant herbs and spices, so it's an easy one-pot meal. It also makes lots of leftovers, which freeze well, so you can choose a larger or smaller roast to feed more or fewer people.

1 teaspoon sea salt

1 teaspoon dried rosemary

1 teaspoon dried thyme

1 teaspoon garlic powder

¼ teaspoon freshly ground black pepper

1 (3-pound) chuck roast

8 shallots, halved

8 ounces baby carrots

2 celeriac bulbs, peeled and cut into cubes

2 cups cubed sweet potatoes

8 ounces cremini mushrooms, quartered

1 tablespoon Dijon mustard

2 cups Bone Broth (page 26) made with beef bones

2 tablespoons coconut aminos

2 tablespoons arrowroot powder

¼ cup chopped fresh parsley

1. In a small bowl, combine the salt, rosemary, thyme, garlic powder, and pepper.

2. Rub the spice mixture all over the roast.

3. Arrange the shallots, carrots, celeriac, sweet potatoes, and mushrooms in the slow cooker.

4. Place the seasoned pot roast on top of the vegetables.

5. In a small bowl, whisk together the Bone Broth, coconut aminos, and arrowroot. Pour the broth mixture over the food in the slow cooker.

6. Cover and cook on low for 8 hours.

7. Top with the parsley just before serving.

A LITTLE LESS PALEO: Replace some or all of the broth with a dry red wine to deepen the flavor of this roast. Syrah, Zinfandel, and Grenache are all good choices that will stand up to the herbs in the recipe, while adding their own spicy flavors.

PER SERVING CALORIES: 552; PROTEIN: 64G; CARBOHYDRATES: 40G; SUGAR: 6G; FAT: 15G; FIBER: 7G; SODIUM: 783MG

Horseradish-Braised Short Ribs

PREP TIME: 20 MINUTES / COOK TIME: 8 HOURS

SERVES 6 Short ribs are fatty and flavorful, and they are delicious when you braise them in a slow cooker. This recipe makes liberal use of horseradish, which adds a peppery bite to the meat and vegetables. You can serve this dish with the broth spooned over riced cauliflower (simply pulse cauliflower in a food processor or grate it and sauté in a little olive oil for about 5 minutes), or with a simple salad on the side.

2 ounces bacon, chopped

4 pounds beef short ribs

1 onion, chopped

8 ounces pearl onions, peeled

8 ounces baby carrots

8 ounces button mushrooms, halved

3 tablespoons freshly grated horseradish

1 teaspoon chopped fresh thyme

1 teaspoon sea salt

¼ teaspoon freshly ground black pepper

4 cups Bone Broth (page 26) made with beef bones

2 tablespoons arrowroot powder

1. In the slow cooker, combine the bacon, short ribs, onion, pearl onions, carrots, mushrooms, horseradish, thyme, salt, and pepper.

2. In a small bowl, whisk together the Bone Broth and arrowroot powder. Pour the broth mixture over the food in the slow cooker.

3. Cover and cook on low for 8 hours, and serve.

A LITTLE LESS PALEO: Make this dish really special by replacing all the broth with a bottle of dry red wine. A Bordeaux works well with this, as does any Bordeaux varietal grape, such as Cabernet Sauvignon, Merlot, or Cabernet Franc.

PER SERVING CALORIES: 741; PROTEIN: 94G; CARBOHYDRATES: 14G; SUGAR: 5G; FAT: 12G; FIBER: 3G; SODIUM: 1,036MG

Argentine Flank Steak

PREP TIME: 15 MINUTES / COOK TIME: 8 HOURS

SERVES 6 The secret to this roast is the flavorful chimichurri, a green sauce originally developed for grilled meat, which you add just at the end of cooking to give the beef savory spice. The flank steak itself is highly spiced, as well, so it's doubly delicious. This is a really easy preparation. Serve it with a side of steamed veggies or a simple salad for a delicious dinner.

FOR THE STEAK

1 tablespoon dried thyme

1 tablespoon chili powder

1 tablespoon coconut sugar

1 tablespoon sea salt

1 teaspoon garlic powder

½ teaspoon freshly ground black pepper

3 pounds flank steak

2 onions, sliced

4 carrots, sliced

1 red bell pepper, seeded and sliced

1 (14-ounce) can chopped tomatoes, undrained

FOR THE CHIMICHURRI

1 cup finely chopped Italian parsley

½ cup extra-virgin olive oil

¼ cup red wine vinegar

¼ cup finely chopped cilantro

3 garlic cloves, minced

½ teaspoon red pepper flakes

½ teaspoon ground cumin

½ teaspoon sea salt »

TO MAKE THE STEAK

1. In a small bowl, mix to combine the thyme, chili powder, coconut sugar, salt, garlic powder, and pepper. Rub the spice mixture all over the flank steak.

2. In the slow cooker, combine the onions, carrots, bell pepper, and the tomatoes and their juice. Place the flank steak on top of the vegetable mixture.

3. Cover and cook on low for 8 hours.

TO MAKE THE CHIMICHURRI

1. In a small bowl, mix to combine the parsley, olive oil, vinegar, cilantro, garlic, red pepper flakes, cumin, and salt.

2. Serve the chimichurri spooned over the steak and vegetables.

PRECOOKING: For extra flavor, brown the beef before you add it to the slow cooker. Heat 2 tablespoons of your favorite Paleo-friendly oil in a large sauté pan over medium-high heat until it shimmers. Brown the meat for 6 minutes per side.

PER SERVING CALORIES: 654; PROTEIN: 65G; CARBOHYDRATES: 16G; SUGAR: 8G; FAT: 36G; FIBER: 4G; SODIUM: 1,116MG

Beef Stroganoff

PREP TIME: 20 MINUTES / COOK TIME: 8 HOURS

SERVES 6 Russian in origin, beef stroganoff has become an American favorite. It features savory beef in a rich and creamy broth. Traditional beef stroganoff is packed with sour cream, so if you're a dairy-eating Paleo dieter, then you can have a more classic version (see the tip). For those who don't eat dairy, however, this version is a tasty substitute.

1½ pounds beef chuck roast, cut into 1-inch strips

2 onions, chopped

1 pound cremini mushrooms, quartered

1½ cups Mushroom Stock (page 23)

1 teaspoon garlic powder

2 cups unsweetened almond milk

2 tablespoons Dijon mustard

2 tablespoons arrowroot powder

1 teaspoon sea salt

¼ teaspoon freshly ground black pepper

2 zucchini, cut into noodles using a veggie peeler or spiralizer

2 tablespoons chopped fresh parsley

1. In the slow cooker, combine the beef, onions, mushrooms, Mushroom Stock, and garlic powder.

2. In a small bowl, whisk together the almond milk, mustard, arrowroot, salt, and pepper. Pour the almond milk mixture over the beef mixture.

3. Cover and cook on low for 7½ hours.

4. Stir in the zucchini ribbons. Cover and cook for an additional 30 minutes.

5. Stir in the parsley just before serving.

A LITTLE LESS PALEO: Dairy lovers, don't despair. You can change this recipe to add creamy dairy. To do so, leave out the almond milk and cook the recipe as outlined above without it. Then, when you stir in the parsley, add 1 cup of sour cream, stirring until it is completely mixed in.

PER SERVING CALORIES: 676; PROTEIN: 36G; CARBOHYDRATES: 20G; SUGAR: 7G; FAT: 51G; FIBER: 4G; SODIUM: 815MG

Beef Burgundy

PREP TIME: 20 MINUTES / COOK TIME: 8 HOURS

SERVES 8 There's no way to make the true beef Burgundy without wine, but you can make a very tasty version by replacing the wine called for in this recipe with more Bone Broth. It's just as flavorful, but it can't call itself beef Burgundy if it has no wine. If, on the other hand, you do use a little wine from time to time, this is the perfect recipe. It's rich, flavorful, and addictive.

2 pounds beef chuck roast, cut into 1-inch cubes

2 ounces bacon, chopped

8 ounces pearl onions, peeled, or frozen pearl onions

4 large carrots, peeled and sliced

8 ounces cremini mushrooms, halved

1 teaspoon garlic powder

1 teaspoon dried thyme

1 teaspoon sea salt

¼ teaspoon freshly ground black pepper

2 cups Bone Broth (page 26)

2 cups dry red wine, such as Pinot Noir or Burgundy

2 tablespoons arrowroot powder

¼ cup chopped fresh parsley

1 recipe Roasted Garlic Cauliflower Mash (page 55)

1. In the slow cooker, combine the beef, bacon, onions, carrots, mushrooms, garlic powder, thyme, salt, and pepper.

2. In a small bowl, whisk together the Bone Broth, wine, and arrowroot. Pour the broth mixture over the beef mixture.

3. Cover and cook on low for 8 hours.

4. Stir in the parsley just before serving over the Roasted Garlic–Cauliflower Mash.

PRECOOKING: Beef burgundy gets a boost of flavor if you precook the meat and bacon. Brown the bacon in a large sauté pan over medium-high heat, about 10 minutes. Using a slotted spoon, move the bacon to the slow cooker. Brown the beef in the bacon fat, about 3 minutes per side (you may need to work in batches so you don't overcrowd the pan.) Move the beef to the slow cooker with a slotted spoon. Deglaze the pan with the red wine, using the side of a wooden spoon to scrape any browned bits from the bottom. Pour the mixture over the beef in the slow cooker. Then, continue with the recipe as written, omitting the wine when you whisk the broth and arrowroot powder.

PER SERVING CALORIES: 738; PROTEIN: 47G; CARBOHYDRATES: 16G; SUGAR: 6G; FAT: 47G; FIBER: 2G; SODIUM: 924MG

Hungarian Goulash

PREP TIME: 15 MINUTES / COOK TIME: 8 HOURS

SERVES 6 This richly flavored beef stew has become a favorite in America. The meat is flavored with paprika, which adds sweetness and a heady fragrance. This dish is traditionally served over egg noodles, but this recipe takes a Paleo turn with zucchini ribbon noodles. To make them, use a vegetable peeler or spiralizer to cut the zucchini into thin strips.

2 pounds beef stew meat, cut into 1-inch cubes

1 onion, sliced

1 green bell pepper, seeded and sliced

1 (6-ounce) can tomato paste

2 tablespoons ground paprika

1 teaspoon garlic powder

1 teaspoon sea salt

¼ teaspoon ground caraway seeds

¼ teaspoon freshly ground black pepper

4 cups Bone Broth (page 26) made with beef bones

2 tablespoons arrowroot powder

4 zucchini, cut into noodles

1. In the slow cooker, combine the beef, onion, bell pepper, tomato paste, paprika, garlic powder, salt, caraway, and pepper.

2. In a small bowl, whisk together the Bone Broth and arrowroot.

3. Pour the broth mixture over the beef and vegetables.

4. Cover and cook on low for 7½ hours.

5. Stir in the zucchini noodles.

6. Cover and cook for an additional 30 minutes, and serve.

NUTRITION HIGHLIGHT: Paprika is a powder made from different peppers in the *capsicum annum* family, which is also the species of chile and sweet peppers. Different types of paprika have different blends, but no matter which peppers are in the bright red powder you use, it's packed with nutrition. Paprika is high in antioxidants, particularly vitamins A and E. It also contains iron and capsaicin.

PER SERVING CALORIES: 385; PROTEIN: 53G; CARBOHYDRATES: 18G; SUGAR: 8G; FAT: 11G; FIBER: 4G; SODIUM: 964MG

Corned Beef AND Cabbage

PREP TIME: 15 MINUTES / COOK TIME: 8 HOURS

SERVES 6 This classic is a favorite in the United States, particularly around St. Patrick's Day. Contrary to popular belief, corned beef and cabbage doesn't hail from Ireland but was created in the United States by Irish Americans. The beef is highly spiced, and the cabbage absorbs the flavors of the beef. It's fragrant when it cooks, and it tastes delicious. If your brisket doesn't come with a pickling spice packet, just use about 2 tablespoons of any pickling spice mixture.

1 corned beef brisket (about 3 pounds), with pickling spice package

1 small head green cabbage, chopped

3 cups Bone Broth (page 26) made with beef bones

3 stalks celery, sliced

3 carrots, peeled and sliced

1 onion, sliced

2 cups peeled and cubed celeriac

1 teaspoon dried thyme

1. In the slow cooker, combine the beef brisket and the contents of its spice package with the cabbage, Bone Broth, celery, carrots, onion, celeriac, and thyme.

2. Cover and cook on low for 8 hours, and serve.

> **PRECOOKING:** Brown the corned beef in a large sauté pan in 2 tablespoons of hot oil over medium-high heat, about 4 minutes per side, before adding it to the slow cooker to increase the flavor.

PER SERVING CALORIES: 472; PROTEIN: 35G; CARBOHYDRATES: 17G; SUGAR: 7G; FAT: 29G; FIBER: 5G; SODIUM: 2,464MG

Asian Broccoli Beef

PREP TIME: 10 MINUTES / COOK TIME: 8 HOURS

SERVES 6 Broccoli beef is a favorite classic Asian stir-fry, and this version is just as flavorful and super quick to prepare in the slow cooker. It has all the spicy, salty flavor of its counterpart, but it doesn't contain all the starch and non-Paleo ingredients you'll get at a Chinese restaurant.

3 pounds flank steak, cut into 1-inch strips

1 onion, chopped

4 cups broccoli florets

1 red bell pepper, seeded and sliced

¼ cup coconut aminos

Juice of 1 orange

2 tablespoons arrowroot powder

1 teaspoon garlic powder

1 teaspoon ground ginger

¼ teaspoon red pepper flakes

2 tablespoons sesame seeds

3 scallions, thinly sliced on an angle

1. In the slow cooker, combine the flank steak, onion, broccoli, and red pepper.

2. In a small bowl, whisk together the coconut aminos, orange juice, arrowroot, garlic powder, ginger, and red pepper flakes. Pour the mixture over the beef and veggies in the slow cooker.

3. Cover and cook on low for 8 hours.

4. Sprinkle with the sesame seeds and scallions just before serving.

A LITTLE LESS PALEO: Soy sauce may bring a more authentic flavor here, if that's what you're seeking. Replace the coconut aminos with an equal amount of tamari soy sauce, and replace the red pepper flakes with a tablespoon of sriracha. You can also add 2 cups of fresh peas (which are legumes) 30 minutes before the dish is done cooking.

PER SERVING CALORIES: 533; PROTEIN: 66G; CARBOHYDRATES: 17G; SUGAR: 6G; FAT: 21G; FIBER: 4G; SODIUM: 162MG

Mexican Beef Stew

PREP TIME: 20 MINUTES / COOK TIME: 8 HOURS

SERVES 6 Beef stew meat is ideal for slow cooking because it cooks best in a moist, low-temperature environment, where it grows more tender and flavorful as it cooks. This version of beef stew has spicy Mexican flavors that make it different from your everyday beef stew, and even more delicious.

3 pounds stew meat

2 onions, chopped

1 (14-ounce) can tomatoes and peppers (such as Ro*Tel), undrained

3 cups cubed sweet potatoes

8 ounces baby carrots

2 celery stalks, chopped

2 green bell peppers, seeded and chopped

1 teaspoon chili powder

1 teaspoon garlic powder

1 teaspoon ground cumin

3 cups Bone Broth (page 26) made with beef bones

2 tablespoons arrowroot powder

1 teaspoon sea salt

Dash ground cayenne pepper

Juice of 1 lime

¼ cup chopped fresh cilantro

1. In the slow cooker, combine the stew meat, onions, tomatoes and peppers with their juice, sweet potatoes, baby carrots, celery, bell peppers, chili powder, garlic powder, and cumin.

2. In a small bowl, whisk together the Bone Broth, arrowroot, salt, and cayenne. Pour the broth mixture over the meat and vegetables.

3. Cover and cook on low for 8 hours.

4. Stir in the lime juice and cilantro just before serving.

A LITTLE LESS PALEO: If you tolerate legumes, add a cup of fresh peas 30 minutes before the end of cooking. For a boozy kick, replace ¼ cup of the broth with an equal amount of tequila.

PER SERVING CALORIES: 786; PROTEIN: 77G; CARBOHYDRATES: 49G; SUGAR: 21G; FAT: 30G; FIBER: 11G; SODIUM: 789MG

Shepherd's Pie

PREP TIME: 15 MINUTES / COOK TIME: 8 HOURS

SERVES 6 Shepherd's pie is a variation of a cottage pie, which is traditionally made with beef. The shepherd's pie is made with lamb, as well as vegetables and, traditionally, a top crust of mashed potatoes. Because potatoes tend to be out on a Paleo diet, this version uses Sweet Potato Mash, which pairs quite nicely with the lamb. To save time, make the sweet potatoes another day and freeze them, thawing and reheating when you're ready to serve.

2 pounds ground lamb

2 onions, minced

3 large carrots, peeled and minced

3 celery stalks, minced

1 teaspoon dried thyme

1 teaspoon sea salt

¼ teaspoon freshly ground black pepper

2 cups Bone Broth (page 26)

2 tablespoons tomato paste

2 tablespoons arrowroot powder

3 cups Sweet Potato Mash (page 50), hot

1. Crumble the lamb into the slow cooker. Add the onions, carrots, celery, thyme, salt, and pepper.

2. In a small bowl, whisk together the Bone Broth, tomato paste, and arrowroot. Pour the broth mixture into the slow cooker.

3. Cover and cook on low for 8 hours.

4. Serve with the Sweet Potato Mash on top.

PRECOOKING: Brown the lamb and onions in a large sauté pan in 2 tablespoons of olive oil over medium-high heat before adding them to the slow cooker. Brown for about 5 minutes, stirring occasionally.

PER SERVING CALORIES: 429; PROTEIN: 48G; CARBOHYDRATES: 32G; SUGAR: 5G; FAT: 11G; FIBER: 5G; SODIUM: 504MG

Rosemary, Garlic AND Shallot Leg of Lamb

PREP TIME: 10 MINUTES / COOK TIME: 8 HOURS

QP

SERVES 8 This recipe uses a butter-flied leg of lamb, which is a lamb leg with the bone removed and the meat flattened. Ask your butcher to remove the bone and butterfly the lamb for you. Or, buy it boneless and put it on the counter with the cut side where the bone has been removed facing up. Hold your knife parallel to the counter and slice into each cut side of the lamb, not cutting all the way through. Then, open the cuts up like a book so the lamb lies in a large, flat slab.

1 butterflied leg of lamb

1 teaspoon sea salt

¼ teaspoon freshly ground black pepper

1 bulb Roasted Garlic (page 33)

3 tablespoons minced shallots

2 tablespoons extra-virgin olive oil

2 teaspoons dried rosemary

1 teaspoon garlic powder

8 ounces frozen spinach, thawed, water squeezed out

¼ cup red wine vinegar

1 tablespoon Dijon mustard

1. Season both sides of the leg of lamb with salt and pepper.

2. In a small bowl, combine the Roasted Garlic, shallots, olive oil, rosemary, and garlic powder. Stir, mashing the garlic with a fork to form a paste.

3. Spread the garlic paste on the cut side of the seasoned lamb, and top with the spinach.

4. Roll the lamb around the filling, tying it with butcher's twine. Put the lamb in the slow cooker.

5. In a small bowl, whisk together the vinegar and mustard. Pour the mixture over the lamb in the slow cooker.

6. Cover and cook on low for 8 hours, and serve.

A LITTLE LESS PALEO: Red wine also flavors this dish really well. Replace the vinegar with a dry red wine. Pinot Noir is an excellent choice with lamb, as is a smoky Grenache or Côtes du Rhône.

PER SERVING CALORIES: 487; PROTEIN: 65G; CARBOHYDRATES: 4G; SUGAR: 0G; FAT: 21G; FIBER: 1G; SODIUM: 546MG

Slow Cooker Lamb Gyros

PREP TIME: 20 MINUTES / COOK TIME: 8 HOURS

SERVES 6 Lamb gyros is fragrant and spicy. You can serve it in lettuce wraps, atop an arugula, tomato, and cucumber salad, or in a bowl topped with chopped tomatoes, onions, and cucumbers, as suggested in the recipe. The dish freezes and reheats well. Divide the gyros into single-size servings and freeze them in tightly sealed zip-top bags for best results.

2 onions, finely chopped

2 pounds ground lamb

2 teaspoons dried rosemary

2 teaspoons dried marjoram

2 teaspoons garlic powder

1 teaspoon dried oregano

1 teaspoon sea salt

¼ teaspoon freshly ground black pepper

Paleo-friendly fat or oil, for greasing

3 large cucumbers, chopped

3 large tomatoes, chopped

½ red onion, finely minced

1. Wrap the onions in a clean tea towel and wring out as much liquid as possible.

2. In a large bowl, mix ground lamb together with the onions, rosemary, marjoram, garlic powder, oregano, salt, and pepper. If you have a food processor, process this mixture on high for 3 minutes or until well combined. Otherwise, simply mix it by hand.

3. Using your favorite Paleo-friendly fat or oil, grease the slow cooker insert.

4. In the slow cooker, form the lamb mixture into a loaf.

5. Cover and cook on low for 8 hours.

6. Serve in a bowl topped with the cucumbers, tomatoes, and onions.

NUTRITION HIGHLIGHT:
Cucumbers are technically a gourd or fruit, although most people consider them a vegetable. They have a high water content, which makes them very low in calories. Cucumbers are a good source of phytonutrients.

PER SERVING CALORIES: 344; PROTEIN: 45G; CARBOHYDRATES: 15G; SUGAR: 7G; FAT: 12G; FIBER: 3G; SODIUM: 437MG

Balsamic AND Fig-Braised Leg of Lamb

PREP TIME: 15 MINUTES / COOK TIME: 8 HOURS

SERVES 8 Balsamic vinegar and figs add a sweet and sour flavor to this savory lamb, which is also liberally seasoned with herbs and spices. Leg of lamb tends to yield a lot of meat, so you can save some in the freezer for future meals, tightly sealed in a zip-top bag.

2 teaspoons sea salt

2 teaspoons dried rosemary

2 teaspoons dried mustard powder

1 teaspoon dried thyme

1 teaspoon garlic powder

½ teaspoon freshly ground black pepper

1 whole leg of lamb, bone-in or boneless

1 pound fresh figs, halved

2 cups Bone Broth (page 26)

½ cup balsamic vinegar

2 tablespoons arrowroot powder

1. In a small bowl, mix to combine the salt, rosemary, mustard powder, thyme, garlic powder, and pepper. Rub the mixture all over the leg of lamb. Put the lamb in the slow cooker with the figs.

2. In a small bowl, whisk together the Bone Broth, vinegar, and arrowroot. Add broth mixture to slow cooker.

3. Cover and cook on low for 8 hours, and serve.

NUTRITION HIGHLIGHT: Balsamic vinegar is made from the juice of Trebbiano grapes. True balsamico from Italy is sweet and slightly syrupy and is made in a solara system, where the juices are moved through different aged wooden barrels and mixed with different vintages of vinegar. For very few calories or carbs, balsamic vinegars can add tremendous flavor to your favorite dishes.

PER SERVING CALORIES: 486; PROTEIN: 51G; CARBOHYDRATES: 41G; SUGAR: 27G; FAT: 14G; FIBER: 6G; SODIUM: 674MG

Peppered Lamb Shanks

PREP TIME: 10 MINUTES / COOK TIME: 8 HOURS

SERVES 4 Lamb shanks are meaty, and because the meat is cooked on the bone, it develops a deep, rich flavor. Lamb tends to have a slightly gamey flavor, but lemon, pepper, and garlic balance it and make these braised shanks rich, tasty, and herbaceous. Each shank weighs about a pound and a half, but you may use smaller or larger shanks.

Zest of 2 lemons

1 tablespoon sea salt

1 teaspoon garlic powder

1 teaspoon dried oregano

1 teaspoon dried rosemary

1 teaspoon dried marjoram

½ teaspoon freshly ground black pepper

2 lamb shanks (about 3 pounds total)

3 onions, quartered

8 ounces baby carrots

1. In a small bowl, mix to combine the lemon zest, salt, garlic powder, oregano, rosemary, marjoram, and pepper. Rub the spice mixture all over the lamb shanks.

2. In the slow cooker, mix the onions and carrots.

3. Place the lamb shanks on top of the vegetables.

4. Cover and cook on low for 8 hours, and serve.

PRECOOKING: To really allow the flavor to penetrate the meat, rub the spices on the lamb shanks the night before. Wrap them in plastic and refrigerate for 8 to 12 hours before adding them to the slow cooker.

PER SERVING CALORIES: 363; PROTEIN: 47G; CARBOHYDRATES: 14G; SUGAR: 6G; FAT: 12G; FIBER: 4G; SODIUM: 1,576MG

Braised Lamb Shanks WITH Orange AND Rosemary

PREP TIME: 15 MINUTES / COOK TIME: 8 HOURS

SERVES 4 Lamb shanks come from the upper part of the front of the back leg. They are best roasted or braised, which pulls all the juices from the bone into the meat. That makes them great for the slow cooker. Here, rosemary has an evergreen aroma that stands up well to the rich flavor of lamb, while the acidity and sweetness of the orange cut through some of the fattiness of the meat. Sweet potatoes on the bottom of the slow cooker soak up the juices and herbs, infusing them with flavor as they cook.

2 teaspoons dried rosemary

1 teaspoon garlic powder

Zest of 2 oranges

1 teaspoon sea salt

¼ teaspoon freshly ground black pepper

2 lamb shanks (about 2 pounds total)

Juice of 2 oranges

3 cups cubed sweet potatoes

1. In a small bowl, mix to combine the rosemary, garlic powder, orange zest, salt, and pepper. Rub the mixture on the lamb shanks.

2. In the slow cooker, combine the orange juice and sweet potatoes. Top with the lamb shanks.

3. Cover and cook on low for 8 hours, and serve.

PRECOOKING: Brown the seasoned lamb shanks in 2 tablespoons of coconut oil in a large sauté pan over medium-high heat for about 4 minutes per side before adding them to the slow cooker. Deglaze the pan with the orange juice, scraping any browned bits (where the flavor is) from the bottom of the pan with the side of a wooden spoon. Pour the orange juice over the lamb in the slow cooker.

PER SERVING CALORIES: 605; PROTEIN: 67G; CARBOHYDRATES: 44G; SUGAR: 10G; FAT: 17G; FIBER: 7G; SODIUM: 651MG

Lamb Osso Bucco

PREP TIME: 15 MINUTES / COOK TIME: 8 HOURS

SERVES 6 Osso bucco uses cross-cut lamb shanks (shanks cut crosswise through the bone in thick slices) that are slowly braised with onions, tomatoes, carrots, and herbs. The tender lamb is then topped with a flavorful and fresh herbal gremolata (a condiment classically made of lemon zest, garlic, and parsley), which infuses so much flavor it's like a taste explosion in your mouth. Osso bucco is Milanese and is traditionally made with veal shanks, but the lamb works here, too.

6 cross-cut lamb shanks
   (about 1 pound each)

1 (14-ounce) can chopped tomatoes, drained

2 onions, sliced

4 large carrots, peeled and sliced

Juice of 1 orange

½ cup Bone Broth (page 26)

1½ teaspoons sea salt, divided

1 teaspoon dried thyme

1 teaspoon garlic powder

¼ teaspoon freshly ground black pepper

½ cup chopped fresh Italian parsley

Zest of 1 orange

3 garlic cloves, finely minced

1. In the slow cooker, combine the lamb, tomatoes, onions, carrots, orange juice, Bone Broth, 1 teaspoon of salt, thyme, garlic powder, and pepper.

2. Cover and cook on low for 8 hours.

3. In a small bowl, mix together the remaining ½ teaspoon of salt with the Italian parsley, orange zest, and garlic. Stir the herb mixture into the osso bucco just before serving.

A LITTLE LESS PALEO: The addition of white wine brightens up the flavors of this dish and adds a hint of acidity. Replace the broth with an equal amount of a dry white wine, such as a Chenin Blanc. You can also choose an acidic white, such as a dry Riesling.

PER SERVING CALORIES: 633; PROTEIN: 87G; CARBOHYDRATES: 16G; SUGAR: 9G; FAT: 23G; FIBER: 4G; SODIUM: 1,426MG

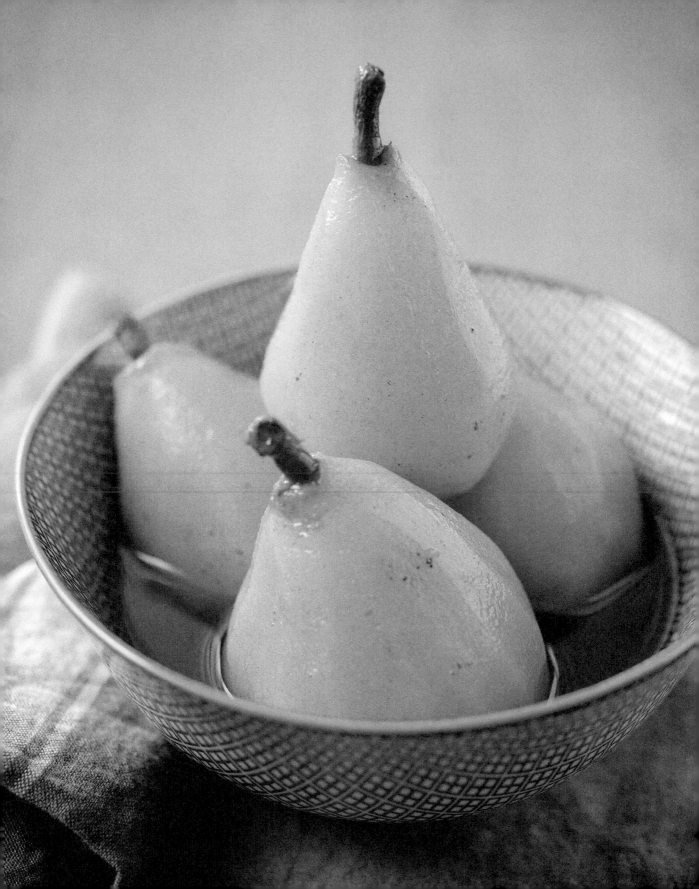

Hot Spiced Apple Cider

PREP TIME: 10 MINUTES / COOK TIME: 4 HOURS OR LONGER

SERVES 6 In the fall, apple orchards fresh-press cider. This rich and flavorful juice is packed with nutrients, and it's even tastier when combined with delicious spices. Keep a pot of this simmering on the countertop all day, and your house will smell great. Not only that, but you'll have a warm treat when you come in from working outside in the crisp days of fall.

8 cups apple cider

¼ cup pure maple syrup

2 cinnamon sticks

3 whole cloves

1 whole dried allspice berry

¼ teaspoon ground nutmeg

1 slice fresh ginger

1. In the slow cooker, combine the apple cider, syrup, cinnamon sticks, cloves, allspice berry, nutmeg, and ginger.

2. Cover and cook on low for 4 hours or as long as 8 hours, and serve.

A LITTLE LESS PALEO: For a boozy version of hot apple cider, add ¼ cup of whiskey or bourbon to the cider before you simmer it.

PER SERVING CALORIES: 190; PROTEIN: <1G; CARBOHYDRATES: 48G; SUGAR: 44G; FAT: <1G; FIBER: 0G; SODIUM: 11MG

Mexican Hot Chocolate

PREP TIME: 10 MINUTES / COOK TIME: 2 HOURS

SERVES 6 So delicious on a winter's day, Mexican hot chocolate is fragrant with cinnamon and a dash of heat from cayenne pepper. This version has added richness because it is sweetened partially with maple syrup. Adjust the sweetness to your taste by adding a little more or less coconut sugar to the final mix. It takes only a few hours for the flavors to blend, but you can keep this in the slow cooker on warm for up to 8 hours.

6 cups unsweetened almond milk

1 (14-ounce) can coconut milk

¾ cup coconut sugar

¼ cup pure maple syrup

6 ounces unsweetened dark chocolate, grated

3 cinnamon sticks

Dash ground cayenne pepper

1. In the slow cooker, combine the almond milk, coconut milk, sugar, syrup, chocolate, cinnamon sticks, and cayenne.

2. Cover and cook on low for 2 hours or as long as 8 hours. Stir before serving.

NUTRITION HIGHLIGHT: Chocolate does more than taste good. It's high in fiber, iron, magnesium, and manganese. It's also an excellent source of antioxidants, including polyphenols and flavenols.

PER SERVING CALORIES: 506; PROTEIN: 6G; CARBOHYDRATES: 46G; SUGAR: 6G; FAT: 34G; FIBER: 6G; SODIUM: 201MG

Maple-Spiced Glazed Nuts

PREP TIME: 10 MINUTES / COOK TIME: 3 HOURS

(LS) (QP)

SERVES 6 Chinese five spice powder adds zip to these sweet nuts with its combination of sweet spices and Sichuan pepper. Maple syrup brings sweetness to the nuts. While the recipe calls for a combination of pecans, walnuts, and almonds, you can use any unsalted nuts and seeds you choose. Remember to avoid peanuts and cashews, which are legumes.

1 cup shelled whole pecans

1 cup shelled whole almonds

1 cup shelled whole walnuts

¼ cup pure maple syrup

¼ cup coconut oil

1½ teaspoons Chinese five spice powder

½ teaspoon sea salt

Zest of 1 orange

1. In the slow cooker, combine the pecans, almonds, walnuts, syrup, coconut oil, Chinese five spice powder, salt, and orange zest, stirring well to mix.

2. Cover and cook on low for 3 hours.

3. Allow to cool completely before serving or storing in tightly sealed zip-top bags.

A LITTLE LESS PALEO: If you absolutely love cashews and peanuts and you tolerate them well, feel free to add ½ cup of each in place of the almonds in this nut mix, or mix your favorite nuts and seeds.

PER SERVING CALORIES: 425; PROTEIN: 13G; CARBOHYDRATES: 17G; SUGAR: 9G; FAT: 37G; FIBER: 5G; SODIUM: 158MG

Berry Sauce

PREP TIME: 10 MINUTES / COOK TIME: 4 HOURS

SERVES 6 This berry sauce is good on any of the hot porridge recipes in chapter 3, or you can have it over fruit, sliced melon, or your favorite Paleo cake or treat, or simply enjoy it by itself. The berries give the sauce a deep color. Feel free to choose any local berries that are available seasonally. Berries are best purchased organic, because they tend to have very high pesticide levels when grown conventionally.

3 cups raspberries

3 cups blackberries

3 cups blueberries

Juice and zest of 1 lemon

¼ cup coconut sugar

½ teaspoon ground cinnamon

Pinch sea salt

¼ cup apple juice

1 tablespoon arrowroot powder

1. In the slow cooker, stir to combine the raspberries, blackberries, blueberries, lemon juice and zest, coconut sugar, cinnamon, and salt.

2. In a small bowl, whisk together the apple juice and arrowroot. Add the apple juice mixture to the slow cooker.

3. Cover and cook on low for 4 hours, and serve.

NUTRITION HIGHLIGHT: All types of berries are nutritional powerhouses, and they also have a fairly low glycemic index, which means they do not cause rapid spikes in your blood sugar. Berries contain high levels of antioxidants, and because they don't raise blood sugar quickly, many people on low-glycemic and low-carb diets enjoy them as desserts and snacks. They are also a good source of fiber.

PER SERVING CALORIES: 148; PROTEIN: 2G; CARBOHYDRATES: 37G; SUGAR: 22G; FAT: 1G; FIBER: 9G; SODIUM: 29MG

Maple-Pecan Applesauce

PREP TIME: 15 MINUTES / COOK TIME: 8 HOURS

SERVES 6 The rich, sweet flavor of maple mixes beautifully here with sweet-tart apples. Choose apples that aren't super sweet, such as Honeycrisp, Pink Lady, or Braeburn. This applesauce is especially good in the fall, when local farmers' markets abound with freshly harvested apples picked at the peak of ripeness.

8 sweet-tart apples, peeled, cored, and sliced

1 cup chopped pecans

¼ cup pure maple syrup

¼ cup apple cider

1 teaspoon ground cinnamon

¼ teaspoon ground ginger

1. In the slow cooker, stir to combine the apples, pecans, syrup, apple cider, cinnamon, and ginger.

2. Cover and cook on low for 8 hours, and serve.

A LITTLE LESS PALEO: Warm, rich bourbon adds a wonderful depth of flavor, and it pairs nicely with maple and apples. To add this non-Paleo tweak, replace the apple cider with an equal amount of bourbon.

PER SERVING CALORIES: 427; PROTEIN: 5G; CARBOHYDRATES: 49G; SUGAR: 36G; FAT: 27G; FIBER: 10G; SODIUM: 4MG

Orange-Cranberry Compote

PREP TIME: 10 MINUTES / COOK TIME: 8 HOURS

SERVES 6 Tangy cranberries and sweet citrus blend beautifully in this delicious compote. Mixing in chopped nuts adds a little bit of crunch to the sauce. This makes a good addition to a tasty dessert or breakfast. It freezes well in single-serving containers, or you can refrigerate it for up to 5 days.

1 pound fresh or frozen whole cranberries

Juice of 2 oranges

Zest of 1 orange

½ cup honey

1 teaspoon ground cinnamon

Pinch sea salt

¼ cup chopped walnuts

1. In the slow cooker, stir to combine the cranberries, orange juice and zest, honey, cinnamon, and salt.

2. Cover and cook on low for 8 hours.

3. Stir in the walnuts, and serve.

NUTRITION HIGHLIGHT: With their tangy flavor, cranberries are one of the lowest-sugar berries. This makes them ideal for adding flavor and color in lower carb dishes or for people looking to keep their glycemic index low for diabetes management.

PER SERVING CALORIES: 189; PROTEIN: 2G; CARBOHYDRATES: 38G; SUGAR: 32G; FAT: 3G; FIBER: 5G; SODIUM: 28MG

Green Tea–Stewed Plums

PREP TIME: 20 MINUTES / COOK TIME: 8 HOURS

SERVES 6 Juicy plums are in season during the summer months. They have a lovely tartness that balances their sweetness. This version incorporates green tea, which adds a delicate flavor to the plums. If you don't take caffeine, feel free to use brewed decaf green tea.

16 plums, pitted and halved

2 cups strongly brewed green tea

¼ cup honey

1 teaspoon ground ginger

1. In the slow cooker, stir to combine the plums, tea, honey, and ginger.

2. Cover and cook on low for 8 hours, and serve.

NUTRITION HIGHLIGHT: Green tea is high in antioxidants, such as flavonoids. It also contains L-theanine, which has been shown to improve brain function, as well as EGCG, a powerful health booster.

PER SERVING CALORIES: 44; PROTEIN: <1G; CARBOHYDRATES: 12G; SUGAR: 12G; FAT: 0G; FIBER: 0G; SODIUM: 1MG

Apples Stuffed WITH Walnuts AND Figs

PREP TIME: 20 MINUTES / COOK TIME: 8 HOURS

(LS)

SERVES 4 To prepare the apples for this tasty stuffing, cut their tops off and use a spoon to remove the cores, leaving the bottoms of the apples intact. Then scoop out all but the outer half-inch of each apple, reserving the flesh to chop up and put into your stuffing. The result will be a fragrant and sweet apple.

4 apples, prepared as described in the recipe intro

6 figs, chopped

½ cup chopped walnuts

¼ cup pure maple syrup

1 teaspoon ground cinnamon

½ teaspoon ground ginger

¼ teaspoon ground nutmeg

Zest of 1 orange

Juice of 1 orange

½ cup water

1. In a small bowl, mix to combine the chopped flesh of the apples with the figs, walnuts, maple syrup, cinnamon, ginger, nutmeg, and orange zest.

2. Stuff the apple mixture into the prepared apples.

3. Place the apples in the slow cooker cut-side up. Add the orange juice to the slow cooker, along with the water.

4. Cover and cook on low for 8 hours, and serve.

NUTRITION HIGHLIGHT: Walnuts are a nutritious tree nut high in fiber and antioxidants, such as phenols and tannins. They are also high in vitamin E and a rich source of healthy omega-3 fatty acids.

PER SERVING CALORIES: 338; PROTEIN: 6G; CARBOHYDRATES: 64G; SUGAR: 49G; FAT: 10G; FIBER: 10G; SODIUM: 8MG

Honey Citrus–Glazed Poached Pears

PREP TIME: 10 MINUTES / COOK TIME: 8 HOURS

SERVES 6 Honey adds sweetness to these mild pears, which become almost creamy when you poach them. For a flavor twist, try different types of flavored local honeys—the flavor comes from the flowers where the bees gather nectar. Pears are in season in the early fall, making that the best time to make this delicious dessert.

6 pears, cored, peeled, and halved

¼ cup honey

Juice of 2 oranges

Zest of 1 orange

¼ teaspoon ground allspice

¼ teaspoon ground nutmeg

1. In the slow cooker, stir to combine the pears, honey, orange juice and zest, allspice, and nutmeg.

2. Cover and cook on low for 8 hours, and serve.

NUTRITION HIGHLIGHT: While honey is high in sugar (it's 82 percent sugar by weight, with about 40 percent of that being fructose), it's also high in antioxidants and unprocessed, making it a more natural, more nutritious sweetener than processed sugars.

PER SERVING CALORIES: 193; PROTEIN: 1G; CARBOHYDRATES: 51G; SUGAR: 40G; FAT: <1GG; FIBER: 8G; SODIUM: 3MG

Maple-Bourbon Peaches

PREP TIME: 10 MINUTES / COOK TIME: 8 HOURS

SERVES 6 Bourbon extract and rich maple syrup make these peaches even more delicious than they are right off the trees. Chopped walnuts add crunch, while citrus juice adds a bit of acidity. Cayenne pepper brings an unexpected dash of heat that's very satisfying in these sweetly addictive peaches. You can also substitute nectarines for the peaches in this recipe, depending on what's locally available and in season.

8 peaches, pitted and sliced

¼ cup pure maple syrup

1 teaspoon bourbon extract

Juice of 1 orange

1 teaspoon ground cinnamon

Dash ground cayenne pepper

Pinch sea salt

1. In the slow cooker, stir to combine the peaches, syrup, bourbon extract, orange juice, cinnamon, cayenne, and salt.

2. Cover and cook on low for 8 hours, and serve.

> **A LITTLE LESS PALEO:** Of course, if you want the real thing, you can add some bourbon to this recipe. Just replace the orange juice and bourbon extract with ¼ cup of your favorite bourbon for a boozy treat.

PER SERVING CALORIES: 124; PROTEIN: 2G; CARBOHYDRATES: 27G; SUGAR: 22G; FAT: 2G; FIBER: 3G; SODIUM: 45MG

Peach Cobbler

PREP TIME: 20 MINUTES / COOK TIME: 4 HOURS

SERVES 6 Most Paleo cooks feel grass-fed butter is okay, as long as you aren't sensitive to dairy. This makes the topping buttery and delicious, which is a nice contrast to the lightly glazed peaches. For best results, freeze the butter and then grate it before adding to the topping.

8 large peaches, pitted and sliced

¼ cup honey

1 teaspoon ground cinnamon

1½ cups almond meal

½ cup butter, frozen and grated

½ cup coconut sugar

3 tablespoons coconut flour

¼ teaspoon ground nutmeg

1. In the slow cooker, stir to combine the peaches, honey, and cinnamon.

2. In a small bowl, cut together the almond meal, butter, coconut sugar, coconut flour, and nutmeg. Crumble the topping over the peaches.

3. Cover and cook on low for 4 hours, and serve.

SEASONAL INGREDIENTS: Peaches are just a suggestion for this cobbler, which is delicious with all types of juicy seasonal ingredients. For example, try a combination of cherries and apricots for the filling, or try the delicious pluot, which is a hybrid of a plum and an apricot.

PER SERVING CALORIES: 317; PROTEIN: 4G; CARBOHYDRATES: 36G; SUGAR: 30G; FAT: 19G; FIBER: 5G; SODIUM: 120MG

Blackberry Crisp

PREP TIME: 15 MINUTES / COOK TIME: 4 HOURS

LS

SERVES 6 Sweetened chopped nuts and almond meal make a nice crumbly topping for this blackberry crisp. Juicy blackberries are best in late summer, when they reach the peak of ripeness. You can also substitute other berries in this tasty crisp, depending on what tickles your taste buds or what is seasonally available.

6 cups blackberries

½ cup honey

Juice of 1 orange

2 tablespoons arrowroot powder

Pinch sea salt

2 cups almond meal

2 cups chopped unsalted pecans

¼ cup pure maple syrup

¼ cup melted coconut oil

1 teaspoon ground cinnamon

1. In the slow cooker, combine the blackberries and honey, stirring to mix.

2. In a small bowl, whisk together the orange juice, arrowroot, and salt. Stir the orange juice mixture into the blackberries and honey.

3. In a large bowl, mix the almond meal, pecans, syrup, coconut oil, and cinnamon. Spread the almond meal mixture over the blackberry mixture.

4. Cover and cook on low for 4 hours, and serve.

SEASONAL INGREDIENTS: Try making this dessert with raspberries in July, or strawberries in June, when they are in season. You can also make it with peaches, nectarines, or plums—whatever is available at your local farmers' market right now.

PER SERVING CALORIES: 734; PROTEIN: 13G; CARBOHYDRATES: 65G; SUGAR: 44G; FAT: 53G; FIBER: 17G; SODIUM: 31MG

Blueberry-Coconut Cake

PREP TIME: 15 MINUTES / COOK TIME: 3 HOURS

SERVES 6 Cake? In a slow cooker? Better yet, Paleo cake in a slow cooker? You *can* make this sweet and moist cake. You can also customize it. Try replacing the blueberries with cherries, chopped peaches, raspberries, or whatever is seasonal and fresh at your local farmers' market.

½ cup melted coconut oil, plus more for greasing

2 cups almond meal

1 cup coconut sugar

¾ cup shredded unsweetened coconut

¼ cup egg white powder

Zest of 1 orange

2 teaspoons baking soda

¼ teaspoon sea salt

4 eggs, beaten

¾ cup coconut milk

1½ cups fresh blueberries

1. Use coconut oil to grease the slow cooker insert.

2. In a large bowl, whisk together the almond meal, coconut sugar, shredded coconut, egg white powder, orange zest, baking soda, and salt.

3. In another large bowl, whisk together the eggs, coconut milk, and ½ cup of coconut oil.

4. Add the wet ingredients to the dry ingredients, folding until just combined. Fold in the berries.

5. Pour the batter into the slow cooker. Cover and cook on low for 3 hours. Allow to cool completely before serving.

NUTRITION HIGHLIGHT:
Blueberries are high in antioxidants, scoring high on the ORAC scale, which is a measure of how well certain foods can reduce oxidative stress in the body. (ORAC is an acronym for Oxygen Radical Absorbance Capacity.)

PER SERVING CALORIES: 509; PROTEIN: 9G; CARBOHYDRATES: 43G; SUGAR: 38G; FAT: 37G; FIBER: 3G; SODIUM: 583MG

Cinnamon Coffee Cake

PREP TIME: 20 MINUTES / COOK TIME: 3 HOURS

SERVES 6 Coffee cake is delicious for breakfast, or it's a tasty treat any time of day, whether you drink coffee or not. This version is made with coconut flour and lots of cinnamon, so it's fragrant when it cooks. For best results, allow it to cool before slicing.

½ cup melted coconut oil, plus more for greasing

2¼ cups almond meal

1 cup coconut sugar

¼ cup egg white powder

2 teaspoons ground cinnamon

2 teaspoons baking soda

¼ teaspoon sea salt

¾ cup unsweetened almond milk

4 eggs, beaten

½ cup chopped pecans

1. Using coconut oil, grease the slow cooker.

2. In a large bowl, whisk together the almond meal, coconut sugar, egg white powder, cinnamon, baking soda, and salt.

3. In another large bowl, whisk together the almond milk, eggs, and ½ cup of coconut oil.

4. Fold the wet ingredients into the dry until just blended. Fold in the pecans.

5. Pour the batter into the slow cooker. Cover and cook on low for 3 hours. Allow to cool completely before serving.

NUTRITION HIGHLIGHT: Coconut oil got a bad rap for many years because it has saturated fat. Recently, however, its reputation has been turning around. Coconut oil is a natural source of medium-chain triglycerides, which have been shown to help produce fat loss when part of a healthy diet, according to the Mayo Clinic.

PER SERVING CALORIES: 397; PROTEIN: 9G; CARBOHYDRATES: 29G; SUGAR: 25G; FAT: 30G; FIBER: 2G; SODIUM: 442MG

Pumpkin Butter

PREP TIME: 10 MINUTES / COOK TIME: 4 HOURS

LS QP

MAKES 9 CUPS Pumpkin butter makes a delicious sweet and spicy spread or dip for fruits. It's also delicious on your favorite Paleo muffins or Paleo pancakes, or you can stir it into a Paleo porridge. This freezes well, so you can make a large batch and store it in smaller containers in the freezer for whenever you want a sweet treat.

8 cups pumpkin purée (not pumpkin pie mix)

1 cup honey

1 cup pure maple syrup

1 cup apple cider

Juice of 1 lemon

2 tablespoons ground cinnamon

2 teaspoons ground ginger

1 teaspoon ground nutmeg

½ teaspoon ground cloves

Pinch sea salt

1. In the slow cooker, stir to combine the pumpkin, honey, syrup, apple cider, lemon juice, cinnamon, ginger, nutmeg, cloves, and salt.

2. Cover and cook on low for 4 hours, and serve.

SEASONAL INGREDIENTS: In the fall and winter, you can use other types of winter squash in this recipe, as well. You'll need to cook the squash first (see the recipe for Spaghetti Squash Marinara on page 92), and then purée it with a blender or food processor before adding it to the pumpkin butter.

PER SERVING (¼ CUP) CALORIES: 75; PROTEIN: 1G; CARBOHYDRATES: 19G; SUGAR: 15G; FAT: <1G; FIBER: 2G; SODIUM: 12MG

Pumpkin Pie Pudding
WITH Dried Cranberries

PREP TIME: 10 MINUTES / COOK TIME: 8 HOURS

SERVES 8 Pumpkin and cranberries are both in season in the fall, which is why they are such popular Thanksgiving treats. Many foodies will tell you, if it grows together it goes together—meaning foods that are in season at the same time and in the same areas make tasty flavor combinations. That's certainly true for cranberries and pumpkin. The dried cranberries add a nice, chewy sweetness to this recipe.

¼ cup plus 2 tablespoons coconut oil, melted, plus more for greasing

6 cups pumpkin purée (not pumpkin pie mix)

2 cups coconut milk

2 cups unsweetened almond milk

6 eggs

½ cup pure maple syrup

½ cup coconut sugar

¼ cup plus 2 tablespoons coconut flour

1 teaspoon ground cinnamon

½ teaspoon ground ginger

¼ teaspoon ground nutmeg

1 cup dried cranberries

1. Using coconut oil, grease the slow cooker insert.

2. In a bowl, whisk together the coconut oil, pumpkin, coconut milk, almond milk, eggs, maple syrup, coconut sugar, coconut flour, cinnamon, ginger, and nutmeg.

3. Fold in the cranberries, and add the mixture to the slow cooker.

4. Cover and cook on low for 8 hours, and serve.

NUTRITION HIGHLIGHT: Sweet-tart cranberries add not only flavor but nutrition as well. They are high in antioxidant compounds and contain good levels of vitamin C, manganese, and fiber.

PER SERVING CALORIES: 473; PROTEIN: 9G; CARBOHYDRATES: 49G; SUGAR: 33G; FAT: 30G; FIBER: 10G; SODIUM: 122MG

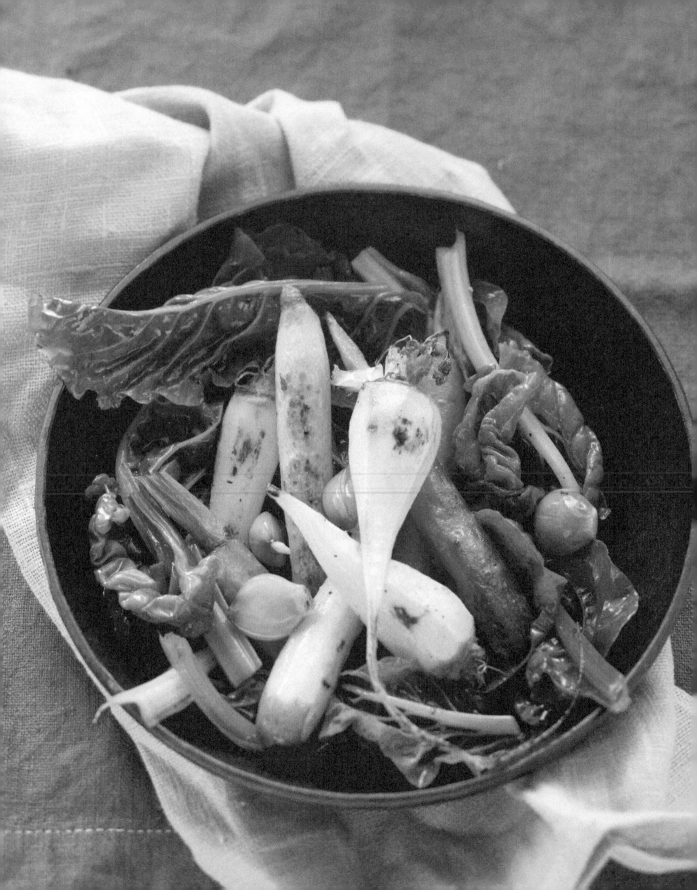

The Dirty Dozen and The Clean Fifteen

A nonprofit and environmental watchdog organization, the Environmental Working Group (EWG), looks at data supplied by the US Department of Agriculture (USDA) and the Food and Drug Administration (FDA) about pesticide residues. Each year it compiles a list of the lowest and highest pesticide loads found in commercial crops. You can use these lists to decide which fruits and vegetables to buy organic to minimize your exposure to pesticides and which produce is considered safe enough to buy conventionally. This does not mean they are pesticide-free, though, so wash these fruits and vegetables thoroughly.

These lists change every year, so make sure you look up the most recent one before you fill your shopping cart. You'll find the most recent lists as well as a guide to pesticides in produce at EWG.org/FoodNews.

THE DIRTY DOZEN

Apples · Celery · Cherry tomatoes · Cucumbers · Grapes
Nectarines (imported) · Peaches · Potatoes · Snap peas (imported)
Spinach · Strawberries · Sweet bell peppers
Kale/Collard greens* · Hot peppers*

In addition to the dirty dozen, the EWG added two produce contaminated with highly toxic organo-phosphate insecticides.

THE CLEAN FIFTEEN

Asparagus · Avocados · Cabbage · Cantaloupes (domestic)
Cauliflower · Eggplants · Grapefruits · Kiwis
Mangos · Onions · Papayas · Pineapples · Sweet corn
Sweet peas (frozen) · Sweet potatoes

Measurement Conversion Tables

VOLUME EQUIVALENTS (LIQUID)

US STANDARD	US STANDARD (OUNCES)	METRIC (APPROXIMATE)
2 tablespoons	1 fl. oz.	30 mL
¼ cup	2 fl. oz.	60 mL
½ cup	4 fl. oz.	120 mL
1 cup	8 fl. oz.	240 mL
1½ cups	12 fl. oz.	355 mL
2 cups or 1 pint	16 fl. oz.	475 mL
4 cups or 1 quart	32 fl. oz.	1 L
1 gallon	128 fl. oz.	4 L

TEMPERATURE

FAHRENHEIT (F)	CELSIUS (C) (APPROXIMATE)
250°F	120°C
300°F	150°C
325°F	165°C
350°F	180°C
375°F	190°C
400°F	200°C
425°F	220°C
450°F	230°C

VOLUME EQUIVALENTS (DRY)

US STANDARD	METRIC (APPROXIMATE)
¼ teaspoon	1 mL
½ teaspoon	2 mL
1 teaspoon	5 mL
1 tablespoon	15 mL
¼ cup	59 mL
⅓ cup	79 mL
½ cup	118 mL
1 cup	177 mL

WEIGHT EQUIVALENTS

US STANDARD	METRIC (APPROXIMATE)
½ ounce	15 g
1 ounce	30 g
2 ounces	60 g
4 ounces	115 g
8 ounces	225 g
12 ounces	340 g
16 ounces or 1 pound	455 g

Resources

WEBSITES

Paleo Lifestyle

MARK'S DAILY APPLE marksdailyapple.com
Former endurance athlete Mark Sisson outlines his take on the Paleo way of living.

THE PALEO DIET thepaleodiet.com
Dr. Loren Cordain offers Paleo recipes, podcasts, and articles.

PALEO LEAP paleoleap.com
An informative website for those just starting out on the Paleo way of life.

PRIMAL DOCS primaldocs.com
A network of physicians and other health practitioners rooted in ancestral health and functional medicine.

ROBB WOLF robbwolf.com
Robb Wolf, a former research biochemist, offers articles and podcasts about Paleo, gluten-free, autoimmunity, and anti-inflammatory health plans.

Paleo Foods and Pastured Meats

AMERICAN GRASS-FED BEEF americangrassfedbeef.com/grass-fed-natural-beef.asp
An online source for pastured animal products that are delivered to your doorstep.

EAT WILD eatwild.com
A terrific database for locating nearby farms and farmers' markets that sell pastured animal products.

LOCAL HARVEST localharvest.org
A directory of local farm stands, farmers' markets, and organic farms.

TENDERBELLY tenderbelly.com
A great place to buy naturally raised Berkshire pork, including pork belly and baby back ribs, all shipped to your home.

DAKOTA GRASS FED BEEF grassfedbeef.com
A good resource for locating pastured animal meat near you.

U.S. WELLNESS MEATS grasslandbeef.com
Home delivery of pastured and naturally raised animal products, as well as sustainably sourced seafood.

USDA DIRECTORY OF LOCAL FARMERS MARKETS ams.usda.gov/local-food-directories/farmersmarkets
The USDA's directory for finding farmers' markets near you.

BOOKS

PALEO FOR BEGINNERS, by John Chatham, Rockridge Press, 2012

THE PALEO DIET, by Loren Cordain, John Wiley & Sons, 2010

THE PALEO SOLUTION, by Robb Wolf, Victory Belt Publishing, 2010

THE PRIMAL BLUEPRINT, by Mark Sisson, Primal Nutrition, 2012

THE WILD DIET, by Abel James, Avery, 2016

APPS

ONLY PALEO, from OOPM Creative, Inc.
Helps you determine whether the foods you are eating are Paleo.

PALEO CENTRAL, from Nerd Fitness
Makes it clear what you can and can't eat on the Paleo diet.

PALEO MAGAZINE, from Paleo Magazine, LLC
Access to the all-Paleo magazine from your phone.

PRIMAL FEED, from Kelly Technology, Inc.
Content from a variety of Paleo websites, including Mark's Daily Apple and The Paleo Solution.

PRIMAL PALEO, from Appy Ventures, Ltd.
Workout ideas and a recipe for every day of the year.

References

Frassetto, L. A., M. Schloetter, M. Mietus-Synder, R. C. Morris, and A. Sebastian. "Metabolic and Physiologic Improvements from Consuming a Paleolithic, Hunter-gatherer Type Diet." European Journal of Clinical Nutrition 63.8 (2009): 947–55.

The George Mateijan Foundation. "Basil." The World's Healthiest Foods. Accessed March 17, 2016. www.whfoods.com/genpage.php?tname=foodspice&dbid=85.

The George Mateijan Foundation. "Ginger." The World's Healthiest Foods. Accessed March 17, 2016. www.whfoods.com/genpage.php?tname=food spice&dbid=72.

The George Mateijan Foundation. "Turmeric." The World's Healthiest Foods. Accessed March 17, 2016. www.whfoods.com/genpage.php?tname=food spice&dbid=78.

Gunnars, Kris. "Maple Syrup: Healthy or Unhealthy?" Authority Nutrition. March, 2016. authoritynutrition.com/maple-syrup/.

Harvard Women's Health Watch. "Foods that Fight Inflammation." Harvard Medical School. Accessed March 17, 2016. www.health.harvard.edu/staying -healthy/foods-that-fight-inflammation.

Jönsson, Tommy, Yvonne Granfeldt, Bo Ahrén, Ulla-Carin Branell, Gunvor Pålsson, Anita Hansson, Margareta Söderström, and Staffan Lindeberg. "Beneficial Effects of a Paleolithic Diet on Cardiovascular Risk Factors in Type 2 Diabetes: A Randomized Cross-over Pilot Study." *Cardiovascular Diabetology* 8.1 (2009): 35.

Life Extension Magazine. "Horseradish: Protection Against Cancer and More." November, 2009. www.lifeextension.com/magazine/2009/11/horseradish -protection-against-cancer-and-more/page-01.

Linus Pauling Institute Micronutrient Information Center. "Garlic." Oregon State University. Accessed March 17, 2016. lpi.oregonstate.edu/mic/food -beverages/garlic.

Mayo Clinic. "Lycopene." Accessed March 17, 2016. www.mayoclinic.org /drugs-supplements/lycopene/evidence/hrb-20059666.

Mellberg, Caroline, Susanne Sandberg, Mats Ryberg, Marie Eriksson, Sören Brage, Christel Larsson, Tommy Olsson, and Bernt Lindahl. "Long-term Effects of a Palaeolithic-type Diet in Obese Postmenopausal Women: A Two-year Randomized Trial." *European Journal of Clinical Nutrition* 68 (3): 350–357.

National Heart, Lung, and Blood Institute. "What Is Metabolic Syndrome?" National Institutes of Health. Accessed March 17, 2016. www.nhlbi.nih.gov /health/health-topics/topics/ms.

Paleo Leap. "Eat This: Bone Broth." Accessed March 17, 2016. paleoleap.com/eat -this-bone-broth/.

Paleo Leap. "The Slow-Cooker: Your Paleo Best Friend." Accessed March 17, 2016. paleoleap.com/slow-cooker-paleo-best-friend/.

Picower Institute for Learning and Memory. "Decoding Sugar Addiction." MIT News. Accessed March 17, 2016. news.mit.edu/2015/decoding-sugar -addiction-0129.

Ryberg, M., S. Sandberg, C. Mellberg, O. Stegle, B. Lindahl, C. Larsson, J. Hauksson, and T. Olsson. "A Paleolithic-type Diet Causes Strong Tissue-specific Effects on Ectopic Fat Deposition in Obese Postmenopausal Women." *Journal of Internal Medicine* 274.1 (2013): 67–76.

Science of Slow Cooking. "Science of Slow Cooking." Accessed March 17, 2016. www.scienceofcooking.com/meat/slow_cooking1.htm.

Simopoulos, A.P. "The Importance of the Ratio of Omega-6/Omega-3 Essential Fatty Acids." *Biomedicine & Pharmacotherapy* 56.8 (2002): 365–79.

WebMD. "Slow Cooker Food-Safety Guide." Accessed March 17, 2016. www.webmd.com/food-recipes/slow-cooker-food-safety-guide.

Zeratsky, Katherine. "Can Coconut Oil Help Me Lose Weight?" Mayo Clinic. Accessed March 17, 2016. www.mayoclinic.org/healthy-lifestyle/weight-loss /expert-answers/coconut-oil-and-weight-loss/faq-20058081.

Recipe Index

Index